NURSING
REVISION NOTES

PRINCIPLES
OF NURSING

S. LAING

30 DUMYAT AVE,

TULLIBODY.

NURSING REVISION NOTES

PRINCIPLES OF NURSING

by
M. J. Jenkins SRN; DN(London); RCNT; RNT; Cert.Ed.; M.Ed.
and
L. Moran SRN, DN(London); RCNT; RNT; Cert.Ed.; B.Ed.

CELTIC
REVISION AIDS

Celtic Revision Aids
30-32 Gray's Inn Road,
London, WCIX 8JL.

© C.E.S.

First Published 1982

ISBN 0 86305 121 9

Printed and bound in Great Britain by
Collins, Glasgow

GENERAL EDITOR'S FOREWORD

The nursing revision series is designed for all nurses in training. The notes are suitable for pre-modular study, post-modular revision and examination revision, and will also be of value to learners undertaking ongoing assessment. While being comprehensive in the major areas of both patient condition and nursing care, they are intended to complement, not replace, existing text books. Each book provides information on basic anatomy and physiology, aspects of investigations and nursing care and practice questions and answers are included at the end of each section. The authors have used their experience in nurse education to select important areas of nursing care for inclusion and I am sure that all nurse learners will find the books of continuing value throughout their training.

AUTHORS' FOREWORD

The aims of this revision text are to help learners:
a Establish their role in the global care of the patient.
b Relate basic physiology to caring for patients so that signs and symptoms of disease processes may be recognized.
c Establish principles of nursing in individual care patterns.
d Be aware of the person in need as a unique centre of consciousness with anxieties, with varying personal and physical abilities and levels of dependence — one who is actively interested in what is happening to him as an individual.
e Test knowledge and understanding of the principles of nursing.
Objectives are set out at the beginning of each chapter. Achievement of the objectives should be tested by answering the questions at the end of each chapter. Do not look at the answers before completing each test. Use textbooks, models and lecture notes in conjunction with this revision text. Make notes in the margin so that you remember to read about clinical observations.

CONTENTS

1 ADMISSION TO HOSPITAL

People usually enter hospitals as patients, as relatives of patients or as visitors. They may have pre-conceived ideas of what hospitals are like, of the attitudes of the staff and of the events that are likely to involve them.

The objectives of this section are:
a To describe the types of admission.
b To describe the procedure used in admission.
c To describe the initial, general and specific observations required.

An individual's pre-conception of hospitals might be the result of a personal past experience, or the experience of others who have been patients themselves or have been relatives of patients. It might also result from information presented by the media as news, documentary evidence, or as entertainment. These pre-conceived ideas in turn affect how individuals present themselves to others in hospital and how they respond to others and to events.

People are frequently apprehensive of hospitals and hospital staff. This is likely to be associated with fear of illness, pain, death, dependency on others, embarrassment, loss of identity and impersonalization. Patients may also fear not being in control of events that immediately affect them and perhaps of not being in possession of all the facts or information about their condition, progress or otherwise that they feel they ought to be.

The nurse should remember at all times that each patient is an individual with his own particular needs. In many cases the person is treated impersonally, and much of the blame for this lies with the condition-task orientated approach to care common in many of our hospitals.

The nurse often sees patients for the first time as they enter the ward doors for admission. Their differentiation began even before this time in the series of events that have led up to the ward admission.

Type of admission

1 Planned

   a) From a waiting list.

Patient has problem(s) ⟶ G.P.

Treatment ⟵ Investigations

Investigations ⟶ Referral for consultation
↓
Investigations
↓
Treatment
↓
Advice
↓
Waiting List
↓
Admission

   b) From another ward or hospital where specific treatment has commenced, having been admitted there from waiting list or as an emergency.

2. Emergency

a The hospitalization comes as a sudden event with little or no time for preparation, either from home or work, via the G.P. or emergency services.

b Via the G.P. or consultant domiciliary visit following a period of illness at home.

c Via out-patient clinic which the patient has attended and where, having undergone medical examination, continuation of treatment as an out-patient is no longer the best form of treatment.

d Transfer from another ward or hospital where the patient has been treated for the same or a different condition.

Therefore, the patient may arrive for hospital admission having had time to prepare himself and his family, having made appropriate arrangements to cover any commitments he has. Conversely, his hospitalization may be so sudden as to render his life in chaos.

Preparation for the admission

It is only infrequently that a patient arrives at the ward for admission completely unannounced. The ward staff are usually aware of a pending admission, which will normally have been arranged days or even weeks in advance, but they may only have been aware of an admission for the time it takes for the patient to go through the intaking procedure via the Casualty/Emergency Department or Admissions Department of the hospital. The admitting nurse will usually be informed of the nature of the admission, i.e. emergency, planned, transfer, etc., the sex and age and name of the patient, and details about his condition.

Taking into account the type of admission, condition of the patient, the probable events that will follow the initial medical examination and assessment and the nature of the care the patient will receive, the nurse preparing for the admission should consider the following:

Location in the ward

Where in the ward will this particular patient be best nursed?

Hospital wards vary considerably in size, structure and general layout. However, most wards have areas where patients can be observed by the nursing staff more easily and more constantly, where emergency facilities e.g. oxygen and suction are more readily accessible for patient care, where special procedures can most easily be carried out, or where most privacy can be ensured.

The immediate bed area

What immediate facilities will be necessary for this particular patient? Depending on the situation, the nurse should ask herself appropriate questions, for example:

The bed

Can the head of the bed be easily removed for suction or intubation purposes?

Has the bed got a firm base for resuscitative purposes?

Can a head-down tilt be achieved quickly?

Is it an adjustable height bed?

Some hospital wards have a variety of bed types while others have not. The newer bed models are multi-purpose, whereas older models need all sorts of additions in order to cope with specific situations.

Additional requisites

These might include:

a Those additions to the bed referred to above, e.g. fracture boards, bed elevators, infusion stands, cradles, bed sides, traction equipment.

b Separate items such as oxygen and suction apparatus, drainage apparatus holders.
c Equipment for special procedures, e.g. siting an intravenous line, taking of blood specimens, passing a nasogastric tube or urethral catheterization.

Events following admission should be anticipated and where possible prepared for.

Documentation

Every nurse will quickly familiarise herself with the routine documents that apply to all patients in hospital, which are usually for hospital administration purposes; and those documents which are specific to the patient and are usually related to his condition, e.g. nursing observation charts, patient assessment charts and nursing care plans.

The nurse should organise her work so that whenever possible she will be available immediately the patient arrives on the ward. Whether she is ready to take him immediately to his bed or whether the patient will need to wait a while, she should greet the patient, introduce herself as the nurse who will admit him, and inform him of the situation as it presents. If the patient is accompanied by relatives or friends, she should enquire whether they are able to wait whilst the patient goes through the admission procedure or need to leave sooner, in which case the opportunity for exchange of essential information between them and nursing/medical staff must be provided.

Most hospitals have developed their own admission procedure; even so, variations can be found from ward to ward. Generally though, most of these procedures incorporate nursing attention to the following points. They have been considered in the order found in the admission section of the daily nursing care plan.

Observations

The term 'observation' is widely used in nursing but may mean many things to many people.

e.g. The patient may be under observation.
    The nurse is instructed to carry out observations.
    The doctor asks for the patient's latest observations.
    Nursing staff keep observation charts.

To observe means to watch, or to note systematically. Observing the patient can be an effective way of gathering information about him, but often the nurse looks, but does not see and sometimes sees, but does not understand or realise the significance of what she sees.

To observe effectively requires a basic knowledge of normal and disordered body function and behavioural patterns and responses. It requires the ability to apply theoretical principles to practice and the ability to relate one sign to another in order to see the whole. The nurse must be aware of the patient's past, present and possible future condition. Observation of the patient begins immediately the nurse meets her patient.

Initial observation of the patient
This obviously includes:
a   Sex, race, approximate age, mode of dress.
b   Position of the patient, chair or trolley-bound, sitting, lying, standing.
c   Posture of the patient, stooped, erect, in need of support.
    Dependency on others, particularly with regard to mobility at this time.
d   How the patient is relating to his environment.
This leads on to:

General observations
These can be made throughout the admission procedure and might include:
a   Level of dependence.
b   Level of exercise tolerance.
c   State of personal hygiene.
d   General condition of the skin.
e   General behaviour, how the patient is responding to events, his state of awareness, his communicative ability.

Specific observations
These are the **specific signs relating to the disease process or condition** which is the probable reason for the admission to hospital. They include taking note of a combination of the following:
Temperature
Pulse
Respiration
Blood pressure
Level of consciousness
Response to stimuli
Position and movement of limbs
Pupil size and reaction
Colour and texture of skin
Presence and description of pain or discomfort
Presence and description of excreta
Evidence of and description of wounds or injury, e.g. bruising, swelling.

Vital signs
'Vital signs' is the term which refers to the signs obtained from the frequent recording/monitoring of:
Temperature
Pulse rate, rhythm, volume
Respiratory rate, depth, character
Blood pressure
The recording of vital signs is especially important in the critical care situation, when fluctuations in the recordings bear greater significance with regard to:
a The stability of the patient's condition.
b The possible necessity for surgical/medical intervention.
c The decision for assistance from life support machinery.
By the time the admission procedure is complete, the observant nurse may be in possession of a wealth of valuable information regarding the patient's condition.
Observations are made and recorded at the outset in order that they can form a base line from which immediate care can be determined, and with which subsequent recordings can be compared.

The urine test
A specimen of urine is obtained from all patients as soon as possible after admission. The specimen is then routine or 'through' tested on the ward and the results are recorded appropriately on the patient's documents. Abnormalities found at this time are likely to lead to instructions to check-test further urine specimens, to save them for inspection, and/or to save specimens for laboratory analysis and investigation.
The results of such urine tests may:
i Give the medical staff a vital clue which may be an aid to diagnosis.
ii Lead to the identification of an otherwise unsuspected condition, e.g. diabetes.
iii Lead to the early detection of abnormalities which allows necessary precautions to be taken during subsequent care and treatment, e.g. emergency administration of anaesthesia to a diabetic patient.
It is essential that the nurse reports to her colleagues if she is unable to obtain the initial specimen for routine ward testing, in order that the next available specimen be saved and tested.
Should the patient be unable to produce a specimen of urine, the nurse should determine whether it is simply inconvenient at that point in time, or whether there is an underlying cause for the inability to void. During an emergency admission when the patient may be shocked or when there is intra-abdominal injury for example, the inability to void carries greater significance, i.e. it might be due to suppression of urine or possible injury to bladder or urethra.

The height and weight
The inclusion of these details will obviously depend upon the nature of the admission, i.e. the condition of the patient, his degree of mobility, the availability of suitable scales to suit the situation.
This information may be required for various reasons:
a Specific drug therapy/dosage may need to be calculated per kilo of body weight or according to body surface.
b Special dietary requirements may need to be calculated.
c It may be necessary to compare subsequent weight recordings to initial weight to determine response to treatment or drug therapy, i.e. reduction in oedema due to diuretics.

Identification
Details of identification, family, social and medical background are usually recorded in the patient's notes at the outset. These details should be checked for accuracy, inconsistencies and omissions with the patient and/or his relatives as soon as possible. This is particularly important when one considers the common practice of transcribing details (usually related to identification) from the patient's notes to various charts, specimen cards and nursing plans or progress reports throughout the stay in hospital.
When such transcribing is necessary, full name, full details of address, hospital number, age, etc. (as appropriate to the particular document in question) should be used. Serious errors have arisen as a result of wrong identity, usually because someone has not followed simple common-sense rules and procedures with the all too common excuse that 'they did not have time'.
The practice of formally identifying patients by asking them to wear identity bracelets varies from hospital to hospital. Certainly, there are arguments for and against the practice. Cries that 'labelling' the patient is the first step to his losing his personal identity, and to a non-individualised approach to care are certainly valid if the 'label' becomes the only means of identifying the patient. It must be emphasized at this point that there is no substitute for talking to the patient in order to determine or confirm identity, the identification bracelet being referred to when the patient's ability to respond coherently or accurately is in question, or when the patient is unable to communicate effectively with regard to identifying himself. The response of the patient to the suggestion of wearing an identification bracelet will depend very much on the attitude of the nurse who makes the suggestion. Usually patients respond favourably when the nurse explains sensibly the need for such a precaution.

Care of property

Many hospitals issue instruction booklets to their patients prior to admission to hospital, giving details of necessary items of clothing or personal belongings that they should bring into hospital with them. Patients may or may not take note of this advice.

This facility is obviously inappropriate in the emergency situation, so the nursing staff are often left with the problem of coping with the patient's property throughout his stay in hospital. Where possible, only those items which are necessary should be brought into hospital.

All excess or unnecessary items of belongings should be given to a relative/friend (with the patient's permission) for return home. Where possible, all patients should be informed of the hospital policy regarding the loss of personal property whilst they are in hospital and of available facilities for safekeeping of personal belongings. All nurses should familiarise themselves with and adhere to such policies and provisions when admitting patients to the ward.

Care of drugs brought in by the patient

The nurse should enquire whether the patient has been taking any drugs at home, whether the drugs have been brought into hospital and whether the patient carries details of his or her drug therapy (i.e. drug dosage card).

There are two issues here:

a The medical staff may have to make a decision as to whether these drugs should be continued, whether a different drug regime be prescribed, or whether all drugs will be stopped.

b Generally, it is the policy that the patient should not retain his own stock of drugs whilst in hospital. This lessens the risk of confusion and possible overdosage when the patient is also prescribed drugs in hospital, and avoids the situation of drugs not being in the safe custody of the nursing staff.

Following completion of the admission procedure, and depending upon the condition of the patient, the nurse should consider the following:

a This might now be an appropriate time for any relatives or companions who have accompanied the patient to hospital to be shown to the bedside. This gives them the opportunity to stay with the patient to see that he or she is settled and comfortable, to exchange information and belongings and to clarify any details regarding the hospitalisation. Advice regarding discussion between the doctors and relatives can be discussed at this time and arrangements made, if necessary.

b Wherever possible, the patient should be introduced to neighbouring patients on the ward and, if ambulant and well enough, should be shown around the ward, the general layout, dayroom/sitting room, toilet and bathroom areas. He should be given appropriate advice regarding telephone facilities, mobile shop, daily newspapers etc. A nurse should not allow patients to miss out on such facilities because they are not aware that they exist.

It is likely that the nurse will have to write details of the admission and subsequent care in the Kardex or Nursing Report. She should follow the requirements of the particular ward with regard to this but should remember the **A B C** of reporting.

A — ACCURACY

B — BREVITY Try to be as brief as you can but remain accurate.

C — CLARITY Use terms that can be understood by all. Avoid abbreviations and use of ambiguous terms.

Admission to hospital. What is the **most likely** combination of items (facilities which

	Emergency — via Casualty, 16yr old boy. Fractured tibia/fibula and minor grazes	60yr old man. Strangulated hernia, 2 day history	23yr old student nurse. Lower back injury	Elderly man who has fallen. Head injury. Very drowsy but restless	45yr old man. Myocardial infarction	55yr old man. Retention of urine	78yr old lady. Fractured neck femur. Thin. Thought to be incontinent of urine	68yr old lady, on long-term treatment for Rheumatoid Arthritis now admitted for Congestive cardiac failure	30 yr old lady. Bleeding heavily per vagina. ?Inevitable abortion
Protective covers for bottom sheet									
Bed with firm base									
Receiver/tissues									
Head-down tilt facility									
T.P.R.B./P. chart									
Suction									
Fluid balance chart									
Oxygen									
Neurological obs.									
Bed cradle									
Cot-sides									
Infusion stand									
Trolley for siting IV line									
Splint/bandage									
Naso-gastric aspiration									
Beams to 'Fix traction'									
Drainage bag holders									
Catheterization trolley									
Ripple mattress									
Sheepskin pieces									
Emergency drugs									
Position — flat 0-2 pillows									
Semi-recumbent 2-4 pillows									
Upright 4 + pillows									

you would consider to be necesary for the following admission situations? Place a tick in each column against your choices. **Answers below.**

	Emergency — via Casualty, 16yr old boy. Fractured tibia/fibula and minor grazes	60yr old man. Strangulated hernia, 2 day history	23yr old student nurse. Lower back injury	Elderly man who has fallen. Head injury. Very drowsy but restless	45yr old man. Myocardial infarction	55yr old man. Retention of urine	78yr old lady. Fractured neck femur. Thin. Thought to be incontinent of urine	68yr old lady, on long-term treatment for Rheumatoid Arthritis now admitted for Congestive cardiac failure	30 yr old lady. Bleeding heavily per vagina. ?Inevitable abortion
Protective covers for bottom sheet	✔	✔		✔		✔			✔
Bed with firm base	✔		✔		✔				
Receiver/tissues		✔		✔	✔				
Head-down tilt facility		✔		✔	✔				✔
T.P.R.B./P. chart	✔	✔	✔		✔	✔	✔	✔	✔
Suction		✔		✔	✔		✔		
Fluid balance chart		✔		✔	✔	✔		✔	✔
Oxygen		✔		✔	✔			✔	✔
Neurological obs.				✔					
Bed cradle	✔							✔	
Cot-sides				✔					
Infusion stand		✔			✔				✔
Trolley for siting IV line		✔			✔				✔
Splint/bandage			✔		✔				✔
Naso-gastric aspiration									
Beams to 'Fix traction'							✔		
Drainage bag holders						✔			
Catheterization trolley						✔			
Ripple mattress							✔		
Sheepskin pieces								✔	
Emergency drugs					✔				
Position — flat 0-2 pillows			✔	✔					✔
Semi-recumbent 2-4 pillows	✔	✔			✔	✔	✔		
Upright 4+ pillows								✔	

2 NURSING RESPONSIBILITIES AND THE MEDICAL EXAMINATION

The doctor may need to examine the patient before the nursing admission procedure is complete. In the emergency situation it is likely that the doctor may need to examine and commence treating the patient as soon as he is put into bed. However, it is often the case that the medical examination follows the admission procedure.

Where possible, the nurse will have anticipated the needs of the doctor with regard to examination and commencing treatment and will have prepared the area accordingly.

The objectives of this section are:

a Pre-examination: Preparation of the patient
                                   Preparation of equipment and area
b During examination: Assistance to the patient
                                   Assistance to the doctor
c Following examination: Care of the patient
                                   Disposal of equipment

Pre-examination

Preparation of the patient

This usually involves two aspects of care:

i An explanation of the examination which the patient is to undergo which is appropriate to the patient's general condition and response and which may be in addition to or instead of an explanation from the doctor.

ii Positioning of the patient. This usually involves:

  a Removal of or adjustment to the patient's personal clothing and to the bed-linen and bed. Whatever the nature of the medical examination, the nurse should ensure at all times the **warmth, privacy** and **safety** of the patient. If clothing has to be removed in preparation for the examination, the nurse should provide the patient with suitable covering. If adjustments to bed, linen, pillows, etc. are required, the nurse should ensure that the patient is as comfortable and as well supported as possible at all times.

  b Placing or helping the patient into the most suitable position for the particular medical examination. One position might suffice throughout the examination but, more likely, changes of position may be necessary appropriate to the type of condition for which the patient is admitted.

    e.g. The patient with chest disease who is breathless may be examined whilst remaining in the sitting position.

The patient with intra-abdominal disease may need to have his chest examined whilst in the sitting position, change to the recumbent position for palpation of abdomen, and then change to the left lateral position for rectal examination.

To avoid unnecessary interruptions during the examination, the patient should be asked if he needs or wishes to do anything before the examination begins (e.g. pass urine) and then be assisted into the most suitable position as near to the time of examination as possible.

Preparation of equipment and area

The nurse should consider the items necessary for routine medical examination:

Stethoscope
Sphygmomanometer
Patella hammer
Torch
Spatulae
Diagnostic set — Ophthalmoscope, auroscope

Also those additions appropriate to the type of condition:
e.g. Items for rectal examination
    i   digital
   ii   proctoscopy (proctoscope, leads, light and battery).
   Items for vaginal examination
   Items for ear, nose and throat examination

Also those items appropriate to any procedures which may be carried out with the examination and which may be a start to treatment:
e.g.   venepuncture — blood samples for laboratory investigation
       siting of intravenous line
       urethral catheterization
       administration of drug therapy

During the examination

Assistance to the patient

Many patients are apprehensive during a medical examination. This, together with the trauma of being admitted to hospital, can make the initial medical examination rather an ordeal for the patient.

Common barriers to effective communication might be the patient's own anxiety, a sensory deficit, e.g. poor hearing, or perhaps a language difference between the doctor and the patient who may find it difficult to understand one another.

The nurse should, therefore, recognise these possibilities and help both the doctor and the patient to communicate with one another.

Explanation of events in the examination as they are about to happen will enable the patient to cooperate with regard to specific responses and position change.

Assisting the patient with adjustments to clothing and correct positioning will enable the examination to be performed smoothly and efficiently.

Assistance to the doctor

The assistance given above will obviously also help the doctor. In addition to the above points, the doctor might need to have various pieces of equipment handed to or taken away from him.

The nurse should, therefore, position herself so that she can be of maximum help and support to the patient. Ideally she should be in a position to offer adequate explanation or instruction to the patient, be able to observe his responses, e.g. facial expression, and be available to assist the doctor if required.

Following the examination

Care of the patient

The patient should be assisted to dress and adjust clothing and his skin should be left clean and dry (e.g. wiped clean of lubricant jelly following such procedures as electrocardiograph or rectal examination). Necessary adjustments to bed and bed-linen are made and the patient is left as comfortable as possible.

He should be instructed whether he should remain in bed, whether he is allowed to eat or drink, and whether or not he can see his relatives.

If the examination is to be followed by further investigations, or if specific treatment is to begin, the patient should be informed accordingly.

Disposal of equipment

Items of equipment used during the examination have to be cleared away and the bed area should be left generally tidy.

The nurse should familiarise herself with the current practice in her hospital with regard to:

 i Transport of correctly labelled specimens to the Pathology Department for laboratory investigation.

 ii Requests for further investigations, e.g. X-rays, blood tests. Requests for further treatment, e.g. physiotherapy and/or requests for further consultation, perhaps by another department in the hospital.

iii Correct method of disposal of the items which are disposable, e.g. used syringes, needles, swabs, speculae, etc.

iv Correct method of cleaning and storing/re-sterilisation of non-disposable items, e.g. proctoscope, leads, light and battery, metal instruments.

Following completion of the examination, if the relatives are still present they should be given the opportunity to discuss the patient's condition, medical findings and prognosis with the doctor. The doctor and the relatives should be afforded privacy in which to conduct this discussion. This should be in a suitable area of the ward and not in the middle of a busy ward or in a busy corridor or waiting room. It is useful for the nurse to be present during such a discussion, so that she is aware of the exact information that has been given to re relatives and is, therefore, in a position to clarify any points that may arise subsequently.

The questions following this section relate to signs and symptoms concerning the various aspects of medical examination. You are advised to answer these questions with the aid of a medical or nursing dictionary.

Practice Questions
Questions on nursing responsibilities and the medical examination
Match the items in column **A** to the explanations in column **B**.

A

a	McBurney's point	**n**	Bell's palsy
b	Kernig's sign	**o**	Bornholm disease
c	Homans' sign	**p**	Café au lait pallor
d	Babinski's reflex	**q**	Choreiform movements
e	Zollinger-Ellison syndrome	**r**	Horner's syndrome
f	Chvostek's sign	**s**	Koplik's spots
g	Trousseau's sign	**t**	Ménière's syndrome
h	Stokes-Adams syndrome	**u**	Osler's nodes
i	Caput medusae	**v**	Argyll Robertson pupil
j	Cheyne Stokes respiration	**w**	Romberg's test
k	Vincent's angina	**x**	Strabismus
l	Dupuytren's contracture	**y**	Petechiae
m	Charcot's joint	**z**	Mantoux test

B
1 White spots on the mucous membrane of the mouth in measles.
2 Marked unsteadiness in standing with the eyes shut.
3 Squint.
4 Abnormally dilated veins that form around the umbilicus in liver cirrhosis.
5 Swelling and disorganisation of the joints in some neurological disorders.
6 Rapid, rhythmic, forceful movements often involving limbs, face and tongue is seen as a motor disfunction in some neurological disorders.
7 Small pupil, sunken eye, drooping upper lid resulting from paralysis of sympathetic nerve in the neck.
8 Inability or resistance to straightening the knee when the thigh is flexed to a right angle, seen in meningitis.
9 Early complexion seen in infective endocarditis.
10 Small painful areas in fingers and toes, seen in infective endocarditis.
11 Corresponds to the area in which the appendix is usually located.
12 Pain in the calf muscles on passive dorsi-flexion of the foot, indicative of deep vein thrombosis.
13 Paralysis of facial muscles on one or both sides of the face.
14 Absence of the pupillary response to light when the accommodation reflex is present.
15 A disease characterized by tinnitus, deafness and giddiness.
16 A rare disorder where gastric hypersecretion and severe persistent peptic ulceration are present.

17 Slowness of the pulse, associated with attacks of unconsciousness due to heart block.
18 Characterized by pain around lower margin of ribs, headache and fever, an acute viral infection.
19 Thickening and drawing together of tissues in palm of hand, causing gradual and permanent bending of the fingers.
20 Abnormal response of the plantar reflex.
21 Ulcerative inflammation of the mouth.
22 Twitching and contraction of facial muscles in response to tapping of the facial nerve, indicative of latent tetany.
23 Claw-like flexure of hand and fingers in response to compression of upper arm, indicative of latent tetany.
24 A skin test which elicits previous contact with tuberculosis.
25 An abnormal cyclical breathing pattern.
26 Small red or purple spots on the skin which may be minute areas of inflammation or small haemorrhages.

Answers to questions on nursing responsibilities and the medical examination.

a	11	j	25	s	1
b	8	k	21	t	15
c	12	l	19	u	10
d	20	m	5	v	14
e	16	n	13	w	2
f	22	o	18	x	3
g	23	p	9	y	26
h	17	q	6	z	24
i	4	r	7		

3 NURSING OBSERVATIONS — VITAL SIGNS

Remember to use textbooks and lecture notes in conjunction with these revision notes. Questions to test yourself are included at the end of the section. Answer the questions in your own words before referring to the answers.

The objectives of this section are to:

a Briefly review relevant physiology.
b Outline the principles involved in making obervations of temperature, pulse, respiration, blood pressure and neurological vital signs.

Introduction

Observation is a term in common use in daily hospital procedures. What do you understand by it? The Oxford English Dictionary defines observe as to 'keep, follow, adhere to, perceive, watch, take notice of by commenting'. All of these activities are inherent in nursing procedures described as observation, and all the senses should be used, i.e. sight, touch, smell, hearing.

To be able to carry out observation of vital signs and interpret the results correctly, the student should have basic knowledge of:

a Physical and social sciences.
b Problems experienced by patients suffering with disease processes.
c Methods of helping patients cope with problems.
d Practice in motor skills concerned with procedures.
e Professional attitudes toward nursing.

Effective observation of vital signs and the interpretation of results are vital to the well being of your patient.

Body temperature

Man is a warm-blooded animal and body temperature remains more or less constant in health. This constancy is maintained by opposing forces of heat production and heat loss. Heat is lost by radiation, conduction, convection and evaporation from the body surface, by vaporisation from the lungs and by micturition and defaecation. Heat is gained by catabolic activity of cells, the activity of tissues, such as the liver and muscles, which generate a great deal of heat, and the secretions of adrenal and thyroid glands.

Regulation of body temperature

The temperature regulating centres are situated:

a In the cerebral cortex.
b In the hypothalamus, which is the main centre of regulation or vaso motor centre.

a Receptors in the skin are sensitive to changes in cutaneous temperature. Impulses initiated by these receptors reach the cerebral cortex and stimulate voluntary responses in the healthy individual to deal with changes in temperature.

b A group of neurones situated in the anterior hypothalamus are responsible for the main control of body temperature. This centre mediates its control via the autonomic nervous system and is sensitive to changes in blood and cutaneous temperature changes. If the body temperature rises, the vaso motor centre reduces impulses to peripheral blood vessels so that vaso dilation occurs. There is increased blood volume in the peripheral vessels so that heat is lost from the body surface by radiation, conduction and convection. Increased stimulation of sweat glands causes conscious sweating so that heat is lost by evaporation. The tone of skeletal muscles is reduced and usually the individual relaxes activity, and attempts to cool himself by removing clothing, ventilating the environment, taking cool drinks and light meals. Body temperature is usually restored to normal by these activities. If the body temperature falls, the vaso motor centre increases impulses to the peripheral blood vessels, thus there is a decrease in the peripheral blood volume, the activity of sweat glands is inhibited so that heat loss from the body surface is reduced. Body activity is increased to generate heat by shivering, the arector pili muscles contract and raise body hair to trap warm air on the body surface. The individual attempts to insulate against cold by putting on clothing, warming the environment and taking food which helps increase metabolism.

Body temperature usually ranges between 36°C and 37°C but there are variations within normal limits. The temperature is usually lower in the morning than in the evening and this is accounted for by physiological activities. If the individual works at night, the reverse occurs.

The processes of growth and development generate heat, thus the temperature of the infant and child will be higher than that of the elderly person. Temperature increases with the secretion of hormones at ovulation and in the first trimester of pregnancy. Temperature rises temporarily when the individual exercises. The temperature also varies in different parts of the body, e.g. skin temperature is usually 0.5°C lower than oral temperature, and the rectal temperature is usually 1°C higher than the oral temperature.

Temperature variation in disease
The constancy of body temperature is maintained by heat production and heat loss and by the efficiency of the vaso motor centre; should dysfunction occur, the body temperature may alter significantly. If the

temperature rises above 41°C or drops below 35°C, and maintains these levels for a protracted period of time, there is risk to the individual.

Fever

Fever is a sign of pathological activity in the body. Direct or indirect stimulation of the vaso motor centre will cause the thermostat controlling body temperature to set at a higher level, so that the normal reaction to increased body temperature does not occur.

The onset of an acute infection is often characterized by shivering, there is vaso-constriction and the person feels cold. The temperature continues to rise to the new setting of the thermostat until the concentration of toxin or pyrogens in the blood begins to decrease. The decreased stimulation of the vaso motor centre causes the thermostat to lower, there is decreased stimulation to peripheral vessels so that vaso dilation occurs together with sweating and the body temperature decreases.

Some causes of fever are:
a Bacterial and viral infections.
b Malignant diseases.
c Allergic conditions.
d Crohn's disease or Sarcoidosis.
e Diseases of the brain tissue or injury to the brain.

Taking and recording body temperature

Principles involved:
a Safety of the patient is paramount. The rules of the Hospital Procedure Committee must be observed. The correct type of clinical thermometer must be used, together with the most appropriate site for recording the body temperature. Age and underlying disease process must be considered.
b Prevention of cross infection is ensured by careful handling and disinfection of thermometer and containers and by providing individual thermometers for each patient.
c Records should be accurate and neat. The temperature reading should be recorded immediately.
d Interpretation of results. Report significant changes in temperature and take appropriate action when problems are identified. Specific management of patients with high or low body temperature depends on the cause of the condition.

The temperature chart is a valuable aid to diagnosis and to the identification of a patient's needs.

Many conditions have a characteristic temperature pattern, as shown in Charts 1, 2 and 3:

Chart 1 shows a classical intermittent fever pattern seen in malaria or more commonly in pyogenic infections. The temperature rises and returns to normal for varying periods.

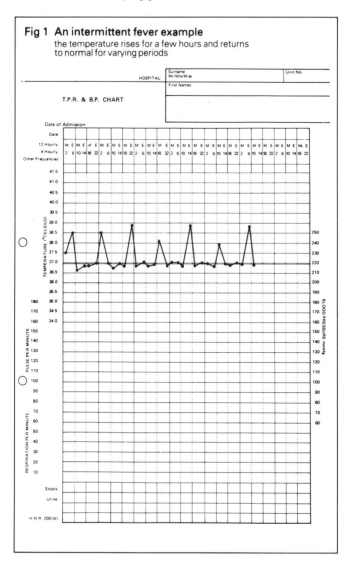

Fig 1 An intermittent fever example
the temperature rises for a few hours and returns
to normal for varying periods

Chart 2 shows a classical remittent fever pattern that may be seen in carcinoma or lymphoma, or when a patient has pus in a body cavity. Temperature drops toward normal but is usually raised.

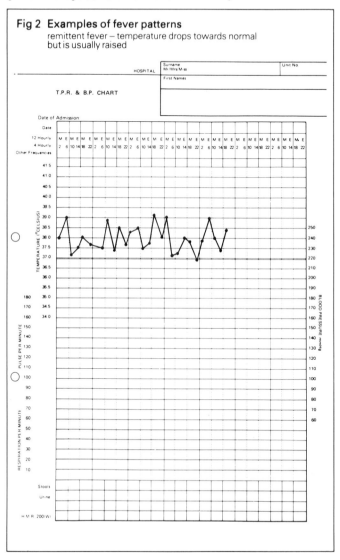

Fig 2 Examples of fever patterns
remittent fever – temperature drops towards normal but is usually raised

Chart 3 shows a classical undulant fever pattern commonly seen when patients suffer with sub-acute infective endocarditis or Hodgkin's disease. There may be periods of fever followed by periods when the fever is not as high.

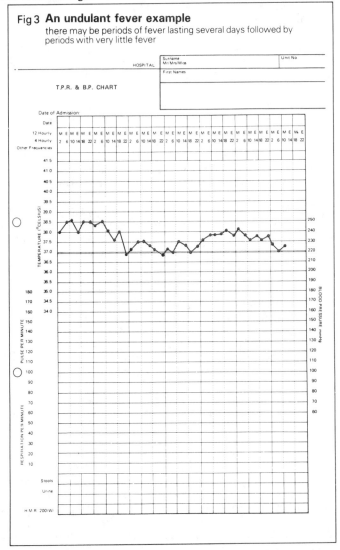

Fig 3 An undulant fever example
there may be periods of fever lasting several days followed by periods with very little fever

Principles of nursing patients with fever

Advise the patient to rest so that body activities are reduced. Steps to ensure comfort depend on the severity of the fever. If the patient is cold, keep him warm but do not apply artificial heat. If the patient is hot, keep him cool but avoid exposure to draughts.

Physical attempts to reduce body temperature include:

a **Ventilation:** Open windows, use an electric fan to make air currents move quickly. Do not expose the patient to draught.

b **Insulation:** Remove heavy clothing, use cool bed-linen (change as frequently as necessary), use a cradle so that sheets are not in direct contact with skin.

c **Cooling:** Pads on the forehead help relieve headache. Tepid sponging helps reduce temperature by radiation and evaporation. There may be a fall of 1°C which will help the patient to feel more comfortable.

d **Giving fluids:** Helps relieve dryness of mouth, corrects dehydration and increases urinary output.

e Observe vital signs as often as necessary and interpret significant signs, i.e. whether the patient is responding to cooling methods or to prescribed treatment.

f Administer drugs as ordered at the correct time. Drugs may be used to reduce temperature or treat infection, or to treat the underlying disease. If antibiotics are ordered, it is important to maintain the desired plasma concentration. The response to drugs should be noted, and side effects identified.

g **Barrier nursing**

If the patient is suffering from a known or suspected communicable disease, he or she should be isolated from other patients and measures should be taken to prevent the spread of infection.

General measures to ensure comfort depend on the level of dependence of the patient. The high-dependence patient will require attention to general hygiene, lifting and moving to prevent pressure, cooling measures, attention to bowels as constipation is often a problem. Unless otherwise indicated, plenty of fluids should be given, of a nourishing type if the fever is of lengthy duration to counteract the effect of increased metabolism. Records of fluid intake and output should be accurately maintained. The patient's general condition should be assessed frequently.

Low body temperature or hypothermia

Low body temperature or hypothermia is less common than fever and may result from malnutrition, blood loss, circulatory failure, lack of thyroid hormone and exposure to cold. Specific management is of the cause.

When body temperature drops, the normal reaction of the hypothalamus is to increase stimulation to peripheral blood vessels and reduce heat loss by reducing the volume of blood in the periphery, inhibiting sweating and increasing body activity. With prolonged exposure to cold, the vaso motor centre becomes depressed, there is vaso-dilation so that heat is lost from the body surface and shivering ceases — therefore, heat loss is not compensated by heat gain. A vicious circle is set up, more heat is lost and eventually the individual becomes confused. Sleep, coma and death result unless the signs are recognised and steps taken to reverse the situation.

Accidental hypothermia
Accidental hypothermia is due to prolonged exposure to cold. People at risk are the young and old. In a cold environment, the very young and the old lose heat more quickly than it can be generated. Contributory factors may be poor clothing, poor house insulation, poor diet, immobility and urinary incontinence.

Management of a patient suffering from accidental hypothermia
Rewarming following accidental hypothermia is done gradually, overheating must be avoided. An intravenous infusion is set up. Blood is taken for haemoglobin and electrolyte levels, abnormalities are corrected and an E.C.G. is performed. Intravenous hydrocortisone and antibiotics may be given. General care includes inspection of the skin for discolouration, attention to hygiene and pressure areas, together with passive exercises. The level of consciousness is checked periodically. It is vital to monitor the temperature, pulse, respiratory rate and blood pressure at frequent intervals following hypothermia during and after the treatment. Cardiac arrythmias may occur and there may be instability of the heat regulating system for a while. Intake and output are monitored and attention is given to the general state of nutrition.

Hypothermia for therapeutic reasons
There are several reasons why hypothermia may be artificially induced.
a   To decrease the rate of metabolism in oxygen use to a part, i.e. a limb with circulatory problems.
b   When interruption to blood flow is necessary, as in surgery to the heart or large blood vessels.
c   To prevent or treat hyperthermia after surgery to the brain, or where brain damage has occurred.
Methods used may be:
a   Application of ice to the body surface, ice bags, ice packs (sheets filled with broken ice), or the blanket method may be used.
The blanket method may be more scientifically controlled than application of ice to the body surface, i.e. the patient is placed between blankets which are electrically controlled and have coils running through

them so that cold water or fluid can be circulated round. The temperature of the water or fluid running through the coils can be controlled by the operator.

b The extra corporeal method. A blood vessel is cannulated, blood by-passes from the patient to an external cooling coil through which it circulates and is returned to the patient via a second blood vessel. A heart and lung machine is used to maintain circulation to give oxygen. Preparation of the patient is important. An intravenous infusion is set up, a urinary catheter is inserted, drugs are given to prevent shivering and to sedate the patient. Thermometers are placed in the oesophagus and rectum and the temperature is carefully monitored. Cooling is stopped when body temperature is within 1°C or 2° C of the required temperature as the temperature will drop slightly afterwards. The pulse, respiratory rate and blood pressure must be carefully monitored together with the urinary output and level of consciousness.

The duration of cooling depends on the reasons for the cooling.

If the patient is unconscious a clear airway must be maintained. Care during and after cooling is similar to that previously outlined.

The heart and regulation of activity
Revise the heart and circulatory system with the aid of models and practice drawing diagrams of the heart and blood vessels.

The heart and blood vessels comprise the circulatory system.

The heart is a cone-shaped muscular organ lying obliquely in the mediastinum between the lungs, more to the left of midline than the right, with the base uppermost and apex below. The heart is divided into four chambers, a right and left atrium and a right and left ventricle.

The structure of the heart in brief
The outer layer or pericardium comprises:

a The parietal or outer layer — a tough non-distensible sac continuous with the great blood vessels and attached to the central tendon of the diaphragm.

b The visceral layer in contact with the heart muscle. There is a potential space between the layers lubricated by serous fluid so that friction and adhesion may be prevented.

The myocardium
The myocardium is composed of muscle fibres known as cardiac tissue, they are incomplete involuntary fibres in close relationship so that impulses for contraction spread quickly through the muscle mass. Impulses do not spread directly from the atria to the ventricles; a ring of fibrous tissue separates them and impulses are conducted through systems of nerve tissue. Heart muscle is adapted to the work it has to do.

The muscle is thinnest at the atria which receive and deliver blood to the ventricles. It is thicker at the right ventricle which pumps blood at a low pressure to the pulmonary circulation and thickest at the left ventricle which pumps blood at a high pressure to the systemic circulation via the aorta.

The endocardium
The endocardium is composed of flattened endothelial cells, forming a glistening lining of the heart muscle; preventing damage to the blood. The heart is divided longitudinally by a septum and there is no communication between the right and left sides after birth in healthy individuals. The heart is divided vertically by valves, on the right side is the tricuspid valve, on the left side the mitral valve. These valves are controlled by fibrous bands rising from papillary muscles; the valves allow the blood to pass from the atria to the ventricles and prevent back flow of blood into the atria when ventricles contract. The pulmonary and aortic valves prevent backflow of blood into the ventricles from the pulmonary artery and aorta. The superior and inferior vena cava deliver blood to the right atrium and the pulmonary veins return blood from the pulmonary circulation to the left atrium.

The regulation of activity — conducting system
The specialised nerve tissues conducting impulses through the heart are:
a   The sino-atrial node or pace-maker.
b   The atrio-ventricular node.
c   The atrio-ventricular bundle or bundle of His, passsing down the septum and dividing into Purkinje System in the ventricles.

The heart functions as a pump delivering blood to the pulmonary and systemic circulation. Events known as the cardiac cycle occur in the healthy adult about 72 times per minute. Each of the cycles takes about 0.8 seconds and involves:
a   Filling of the atria(when the a/v valves are open). When the atria are full the sino-atrial node is stimulated by the autonomic system; the atria contract forcing blood into the ventricles; this is known as atrial systole and takes 0.1 sec.
b   The stretched ventricles contract as the impulses are passed from the wave of excitation created in the atria, from the a/v node to the bundle of His and Purkinje fibres. The atrio-ventricular valves are closed. The pressue in the ventricles exceeds the pressure in the aorta and pulmonary artery, their valves open and blood is forced through. This is known as ventricular systole and takes 0.3 sec.
c   **a** and **b** are followed by relaxation of the atria and ventricles. This is known as diastole and takes 0.4 sec.

Nervous regulation of the heart is mediated from the cardiac inhibiting and accelerating centre in the medulla oblongata. Para sympathetic impulses via the vagus or tenth cranial nerve slow down and strengthen the heart rate. Sympathetic impulses from the cervical ganglion increase the rate of contraction. In health the vagus nerve is dominant. Chemoreceptors in the great vessels monitor changes in pH and blood pressure and convey messages to the cardiac centre. An increase in blood pressure brings about a slowing of heart rate. A rise in carbon dioxide PCO_2 and decrease in oxygen P_2 in the blood will bring about an increase in heart rate.

The rate and force of the heart is influenced by alterations in the electrolytes. An excess of potassium (K) causes abnormalities in conduction and contraction and may lead to cardiac arrest. An excess of calcium strengthens and prolongs systole, lack of calcium prolongs diastole. Low PO_2 results in weakening of heart muscle, while excess PCO_2 impairs conduction and contractility of heart muscle. When the heart functions are affected by changes, characteristic alterations occur in the rate, rhythm, volume and tension of the pulse which can be observed when the pulse is palpated.

The arterial pulse

Pulsation in arteries results from pressure changes within the arterial system. With each contraction of the heart blood is forced into the aorta causing a rise in blood pressure and expansion of the artery. During diastole blood is forced on through the arterial system by recoil and relaxation of the elastic arteries, setting up a fluid wave which is transmitted through the arterial walls and blood to the peripheral arteries. The speed of pulse wave is dependent on the condition of the arteries. Pulsation is less marked in small arteries and is lost completely in the capillaries.

The pulse rate

The healthy infant has a fast pulse rate between 100-140 beats per minute. The rate slows as the child grows and by puberty the pulse reaches adult rate in the region of 70-80 beats per minute. The pulse rate of an adult may range between 50-88 beats per minute. Athletes may have a resting pulse rate of 40-50 beats per minute.

The rate of pulse slows with rest in health and is usually slowest when the individual is asleep. The sleeping pulse rate is a valuable observation when tachycardia may be thought to be due to emotion or exercise. The rate of the pulse increases with exercise and emotion. Overindulgence in coffee, cigarettes and alcohol may increase the pulse rate. Tachycardia describes an increase in pulse rate from normal. Bradycardia describes a slower pulse rate than normal.

Tachycardia is an important feature of bleeding in shock, thyrotoxicosis and fever. Bradycardia is an important feature in heartblock, obstructive jaundice, hypothyroidism and raised intracranial pressure.

Pulse rhythm
Pulse rhythm describes the regularity of intervals between pulsations.

Abnormalities of rhythm
Extra systole is a common form of irregular heart action. It is characterised by a premature beat followed by a pause and a more forceful heart beat. Extra systole may be associated with over-indulgence in smoking and taking coffee and tea. With increasing age extra systoles may indicate underlying heart disease.

Paroxysmal tachycardia
This may occur at any age. The pulse rate may increase to 160 beats per minute as ectopic foci take over the function of the pacemaker and rapid impulses may be discharged from the atria, a/v node or ventricles. The attacks may last seconds or hours and may suddenly cease. Sinus rhythm is usually restored but extra systoles may occur. In later years thyrotoxicosis or coronary artery disease may be the cause. Atrial flutter is less common and is associated with coronary or hypertensive heart disease. Ectopic foci in the atria may discharge between 200-300 impulses per minute. The ventricles are unable to cope with the output of impulses and respond only to every 3rd or 4th atrial contraction. Halving or doubling of the pulse rate is characteristic of flutter.

Atrial fibrillation
This is a common arrhythmia. The atrial muscle bundles contract independently at a rate of 400-500 beats per minute. There is inco-ordination between the atria and ventricles. The pulse is characteristically irregular in force and rhythm.

Heart block
This may occur in three degrees of severity, and is a less common type of arrhythmia, frequently associated with coronary artery disease or overdose of digoxin. Complete heart block is characterised by very regular and slow pulse beats that occur when the ventricles contract independently of the atria.

The pulse rate in shock, excepting vasovagal shock, is rapid and may be weak and thready. The pulse, when bleeding is evident or suspected, is rapid and will continue to increase in rate. It may be of poor volume, there is usually pallor, sweating, air hunger and hypotension. Pulse volume and tension may be estimated by palpating the pulse. A more accurate assessment is made by using a sphygmomanometer. Volume indicates the strength of the heart contraction and tension indicates the state of the arteries.

Taking and recording the pulse
Information to be obtained from palpating the pulse is relevant to the state of the heart and the arteries. In young people arteries are soft and easily compressed. Degeneration with age results in thickening and hardening; arteries feel whiplike.
Diseases of the heart give rise to characteristic alterations in sinus rhythm.
The pulse is palpated most easily when an artery passes superficially over a bone. The site most commonly used for taking the pulse of an adult is at the radial artery, but other convenient sites are the facial, temporal, carotid or femoral arteries.

Principles to be observed when taking the pulse.
1 The individual must be at rest.
2 The most appropriate site for palpating the pulse should be chosen. Two fingers should be placed over the site of the pulse chosen, the pulse should be monitored for one minute. If underlying heart disease is present significant alterations may occur in the space of a minute which may not be noted if the pulse is monitored for only thirty seconds.
3 The frequency of recording depends on the state of the patient and may be daily, twice daily, 4 hourly, hourly or half hourly.
4 Recordings should be compared with a base line and significant changes in rate, rhythm or volume should be reported. Neat records should be made immediately.
5 It will probably be more effective to count the heartbeats of a young infant with a stethoscope than to try to palpate the pulse. In diseases of the heart such as atrial fibrillation the apex and radial heart beats are counted simultaneously by two people, and the difference between the heart rate and pulse rate is calculated and noted. There is usually a significant difference between the beats recorded at the apex and radial pulse.

All the vital signs are usually recorded together unless specific requests for pulse recordings are made. The general reaction of the patient is assessed, alteration in colour is observed, as are any signs of pain or discomfort. The patient's needs are identified and dealt with if possible. Patients with acute heart conditions are usually very anxious. Try not to alarm the patient if significant abnormalities are noted. Chart and report abnormal finds immediately.

Respiration

There are two phases involved in respiration, they are:

a Internal respiration which describes the process of osmosis and diffusion between cells and tissue fluid, which enables the cells to obtain nutrients and oxygen and to excrete waste products.

b External respiration describes the process by which gases are taken into and excreted from the lungs. Gases are interchanged between the capillaries surrounding the alveoli and the air in the alveoli. To remain healthy, the individual has to effect a constant exchange of oxygen and carbon dioxide with the environment.

Mechanism of external respiration

The structures involved are the upper and lower respiratory tracts, thorax, diaphragm, intercostal muscles and nerves.

The sequence of respiration is rhythmical in health, i.e. inspiration, expiration, pause. The respiratory rate is influenced by age, health, emotion, exercise. At rest the adult breathes at a rate of 14-20 respirations per minute. Oxygen reaches the lungs through inspiration of air, and carbon dioxide and water are excreted to the atmosphere by expiration.

Inspiration occurs as a result of muscular effort. The ribs move up and out and the diaphragm contracts, the size of the thorax is increased by three dimensions. The parietal pleura, in close association with the ribs, moves out and the visceral pleura follows. The elastic tissue enables the lungs to stretch, as do the bronchi and bronchioles, letting air in to mix with the residual air in the alveoli. Pressures in the lungs during inspiration are below atmospheric pressures (760 mmHg at sea level).

Expiration occurs as a result of passive movements as all the structures involved in respiration assume their natural positions. Thus all air is squeezed out, apart from the residual volume.

Exchange of gases in the lungs

The gas molecules of oxygen and carbon dioxide set up ceaseless movements and exert pressure on the walls of the alveoli and capillaries. Gases tend to diffuse from an area of higher pressure to an area of lower pressure. The partial pressures of oxygen and carbon dioxide in the alveoli are 100 mmHg and 38 mmHg respectively; when the partial pressure of oxygen and carbon dioxide in the capillaries going to the alveoli are 40 mmHg and 44 mmHg respectively, oxygen diffuses from the alveoli into the capillaries and carbon dioxide diffuses from the capillaries into the alveoli. Oxygen, carbon dioxide and nitrogen in inspired air have values of 20%, 0.04% and 79% respectively. In expired air the values change to 16%, 4%, nitrogen remains the same and water vapour and bacteria are also excreted.

Movement of air in and out of the lungs
Movement of air in and out of the lungs depends on the depth of breathing, exercise, emotion and stress, and the health of the individual. The terms used to discuss movement of air are:

Tidal volume	Residual volume	Inspiratory residual volume	Expiratory residual volume
500 mls in quiet breathing	1500 mls always left in	1500 mls on forced inspiration	1500 mls on forced expiration

The vital capacity is the volume of air that can be expelled by the deepest possible expiration after the deepest possible inspiration.
The vital capacity of a healthy young man is about 4—4.6 litres.

Respiratory function tests
Respiratory function tests are important in estimating the respiratory ability of an individual and are used frequently to assess individuals who suffer with obstructive airway conditions. Various types of spirometers are used to carry out these tests.

1 **Vital capacity tests.** Normal values equal about 4,000-5,000 mls. The patient is asked to breathe in deeply, then to breathe out forcefully into a spirometer. The volume is measured, less than 3,000 ml recorded indicates respiratory insufficiency.

2 **Timed vital capacity test.** The volume of air exhaled into a spirometer as rapidly as possible after deep inspiration is timed at 1,2 and 3 second intervals, and the volume is measured. T.V.C. is reduced in chronic obstructive disease of the airways. This test can cause some distress to patients with respiratory insufficiency.

3 **Minute volume** is obtained by measuring the volume of ventilation in one minute. The total volume is measured with a spirometer and multiplied by the number of respirations per minute; normal values are about 6,000 ml.

4 **Forced expiratory capacity.** This is a timed test measured with a spirometer, the person is asked to breathe out as quickly as they can after taking a deep breath in. Reduction in forced expiratory capacity indicates some expiratory obstruction.

5 **Broncho-spirometry.** This test determines separately each lung capacity and the gaseous exchange between the aveoli and blood. This is a more complicated test than test **4** and involves passing a double lumen tube via the trachea into each bronchus; each lung function is measured separately. Recordings are made on the spirometer. The preparation of the patient involves obtaining permission, an explanation is given and preparation for local anaesthetic is made. After care is as for patients undergoing bronchoscopy.

6 Blood tests include:

a Blood gases analysis
b Erythrocyte and white cell count (total differential)
c Haemoglobin

7 Chest X-Ray.

Control mechanisms of respiration — nervous and chemical
Nervous control
A group of neurones situated in the medulla oblongata composes the respiratory centre.The neurones are thought to be sensitive to afferent impulses initiated by expiration. The respiratory centre, when stimulated, sends out impulses to the spinal cord. These are transmitted to the diaphragm by the phrenic nerves and to the intercostal muscles by the intercostal nerve, thus the inspiration cycle starts.

Chemical control
Chemoreceptors in the large arteries are sensitive to a lack of oxygen and excess of carbon dioxide. If PCO_2 rises and PO_2 decreases, impulses are conveyed to the respiratory centre and the respiratory rate increases. In chronic respiratory disease, PCO_2 is above normal limits and provides stimulation for the respiratory centre. If too high a volume or percentage of oxygen is given in treatment, the stimulus will be removed and a vicious circle is set up:
a Respiration is depressed
b PCO_2 is retained
c Respiratory acidosis occurs
d Mental disturbance occurs
e Coma and death result, if events are not recognised.
Respiration is necessary for:
a Existence
b Maintenance of pH of body fluids
c Voice production
d Aiding venous return by suction on great veins

Recording the respiratory rate
The respiratory rate varies with size, age, activity and health of the individual; various drugs influence respiratory rate.

Normal ranges
The healthy infant respiratory rate may range between 25 and 35 per minute. The rate slows as the child grows. Adult respiratory rates vary between 14 and 20 respirations per minute. The respiratory rate slows with sleep and increases with exercise, emotion or excitement.
Taking the respiratory rate involves counting the rise and fall of the chest as one respiration. The character and rhythm should be noted and

counted for one minute. Any abnormal manifestations such as cough, pain, wheezing and abnormal chest movements should be reported, together with alteration in colour.

Types of respiration characteristic of disease

a Pleurisy and pneumonia respirations are usually rapid and shallow, and accompanied by pain.

b Respiratory acidosis is characterized by very deep breathing.

c Cheyne Stokes respirations, e.g. in cardiac or respiratory diseases, are characterized by hyperpnoea or deep breathing. This reduces PCO_2 level, the respiratory centre is depressed and cessation of breathing occurs. The PCO_2 builds up and the cycle starts again. This is repeated about every three minutes.

d Dyspnoea usually accompanies heart and lung conditions and describes difficult and laborious breathing.

Management of persons with respiratory problems

Efforts are directed towards helping the patient cope with his disease. The most appropriate measures should be employed to help him breathe more easily. Respiratory disturbances can be very frightening to the patient and his or her fear can be exacerbated by lack of explanation and lack of reassurance that such fears are recognised.

If drugs or oxygen therapy are used to treat or relieve the condition, observation of the patient's response to the treatment must be made. Observation of vital signs should be made as frequently as necessary, together with observation of colour and complaints of pain. Significant changes should be noted and reported verbally and in the Kardex.

Blood pressure

Blood pressure is commonly described as the force which blood exerts on the blood vessel walls.

Blood pressure is highest in the large arteries and lowest in the great veins.

Arterial blood pressure

The rise and fall of pressure within the arteries depends on cardiac output. The height of blood pressure depends on the cardiac output and peripheral resistance set up by the arterioles.

The highest pressure in the arteries in the healthy adult ranges between 110-130 mmHg and is known as the systolic pressure. The lowest pressure in the arteries in the healthy adult ranges between 70-88 mmHg and is known as the diastolic pressure. The difference between the systolic and diastolic pressure is called the pulse pressure.

With each contraction of the healthy heart, about 70 mls of blood is ejected into the aorta which expands and the blood pressure rises in the arteries. During ventricular relaxation blood is forced on by recoil and relaxation of the arteries which, by their elasticity, help maintain the flow of blood. Little resistance to the flow of blood is offered by these arteries. The metarterioles and arterioles set up a resistance to the flow of blood by maintaining a state of partial contraction and this determines the rate of blood flow through the capillaries. This is known as peripheral resistance, important in maintaining blood pressure within normal limits. The control of arterioles is mediated by chemical and autonomic control.

Factors affecting blood pressure
These are:
1   The force of the heart action and output of blood.
2   The volume and viscosity of blood in circulation.
3   The elasticity of arteries and the resistance of the peripheral arterioles.
4   Venous return.

The **force** of the heart action and cardiac output will be determined by the state of the heart and venous return. If the heart muscle is damaged, or if there is a reduction in venous return, the pressure and volume of blood ejected with each ventricular contraction will be reduced and the arterial blood pressure will drop, e.g. as in myocardial infarction, or reduction in blood volume from shock or haemorrhage.

The rise in blood pressure which occurs with exercise or emotion is due to increased cardiac output and possibly reduced resistance. The blood pressure returns to normal when the individual is rested or calm.

Aldosterone increases blood pressure by promoting absorption of sodium by the kidney tubules. The increased sodium concentration in blood causes the absorption of more water by the kidney tubules and increases the total vascular volume. A decrease in absorption of aldosterone causes a lowering of blood pressure.

The **elasticity** of arteries in youth tends to diminish with age. The pulse pressure increases and the systolic pressure will rise. In the condition known as essential hypertension, the cardiac output is normal but the peripheral resistance is increased.

The **arterioles** are usually in a state of partial contraction so that blood pressure is maintained. The size of the arteries is controlled by chemicals in the extracellular fluid and by the autonomic nervous system.

If the arterioles are in a state of relaxation, more blood will circulate to the capillaries and the blood pressure may remain within normal limits or drop to below normal. If the arterioles are in a state of contraction, less blood will circulate to the capillaries and the blood pressure may remain within normal limits or rise above normal. The nerves which maintain the tone of vessels are vaso constrictors and vaso dilators, and impulses are delivered to the smooth muscles of the vessels from the vaso motor centre in the medulla oblongata, and some impulses may arise from the spinal cord. Impulses to the blood vessels from the vaso motor centre are stimulated by impulses received from, e.g. blood vessels, pressoreceptors in the skin and muscles and chemoreceptors.

Chemicals and hormones affect the blood vessels, e.g. increased PCO_2 and decreased PO_2 lead to vaso constriction and increased resistance. Histamine released from damaged cells is a strong vaso dilator. Renin secreted by kidney tissue causes vaso constriction.

Viscosity of blood is dependent on the plasma protein levels and numbers of red cells in circulation. Viscosity changes when there is increase or decrease in red cells or when blood is diluted.

Measurement of blood pressure

Principles involved

The individual must be at rest physically and calm, as anxiety may cause a transient rise in blood pressure. Usually, the blood pressure is taken in the right arm, except when there is an obvious reason for taking it in the left arm.

Ensure the cuff of the sphygmomanometer is evenly applied on the upper arm so that the brachial artery can be palpated easily, attach the cuff tube to the sphygmomanometer (which should be on a level with the patient), quickly inflate the cuff so that the presssure constricts the artery, place the stethoscope over the brachial artery and slowly reduce pressure in the cuff. The systolic pressure is usually taken as the point where sounds reappear as the pressure over the artery is relieved. The diastolic pressure is recorded at the lowest point heard through the stethoscope. (It is important to adhere to the advice of the Procedure Committee regarding the last point, as some consider the diastolic pressure recording should be taken at the point where there is a change from loud to muffled sounds.) Remove the sphygmomanometer cuff and record the readings on the chart, significant changes should be reported verbally.

Variations in blood pressure

Health, age, activity, emotion and weight have a bearing on blood pressure. In the infant and the young child, the blood pressure varies between 50–90 mmHg systolic and 40–50 mmHg diastolic. This increases with age until the period around puberty when the blood pressure reaches, within normal healthy limits of an adult, between 110–130 mmHg systolic and 70–88 mmHg diastolic. With the decrease in elasticity of the arteries in middle life, the systolic pressure and later diastolic pressure rises. It is difficult to state the normal and abnormal pressures for an individual, as one person may be able to tolerate high pressure for an individual, that would make another person ill. However, a diastolic pressure of 90 mmHg reached in middle life is usually considered to be reasonable. Factors which cause transitory rises in blood pressure are fear, anxiety, tension and excitement, when there is vaso constriction causing the increase.

Exercise causes an increased venous return with increased force of contraction and cardiac output, causing the systolic blood pressure to rise. The blood pressure returns to normal when the individual rests. Hypertension describes high blood pressure and hypotension describes low blood pressure.

Hypertension
1 Hypertension may be due to increased peripheral resistance and decreased elasticity of the arteries (essential hypertension accounts for 80% of patients in this group).
2 Hypertension associated with renal disease.
3 Hypertension associated with endocrine disease.
4 Hypertension associated with coarctation of the aorta.
Treatment depends on the cause.

Use of drugs in treatment of hypertension
Diuretics are usually given initially, e.g. Frusemide 40–120 mgms daily or a combination of hypotensive drugs and diuretics may be used. Examples of drugs available that lower blood pressure are the sympathetic blocking agents and the ganglion blocking agents. When treatment is started, the blood pressure is usually recorded four times daily. The aim is to lower the blood pressure to a level the patient can live with comfortably. With sympathetic blocking agents, there may be swings in the blood pressure until the patient is stabilized. The ganglion blocking agents have many side effects such as postural hypotension, so blood pressure readings have to be taken while the patient is standing and lying. There may be constipation, difficulty with micturition or visual disturbances associated with drug treatment.
The blood pressure must be monitored carefully during the stabilization period. The recordings are made in different colours on the chart, indicating the standing and lying position. During the standing recording, the patient should be positioned near the bed in case he has postural hypotension and faints. The general reaction of the patient is observed, i.e. whether headaches are experienced or dryness of mouth, and whether complaints of constipation are made. Unexpected manifestations should be reported. The patient's problems should be identified and dealt with if possible.

Hypotension

Hypotension, or low blood pressure, may be due to many causes. For example, it is a feature of myxoedema and Addison's disease. It may be associated with drug treatment of hypertension, or it may be due to shock. Neurogenic shock is associated with pain, fear, bad news or trauma. Vasodilatation occurs with a subsequent drop in blood pressure, the patient may faint. Hypovolaemic shock indicates that body fluids have been lost as in haemorrhage, burns or dehydration, or there may have been increased vaso dilatation when blood becomes pooled in the muscles so that blood volume is decreased.

Treatment is of the cause. If the patient is shocked, the blood pressure together with all the vital signs must be recorded frequently. Systolic blood pressure of less than 100 mmHg over a period of time causes serious oxygen deficiencies in the tissues and reversible shock may become irreversible shock as compensatory mechanisms fail. The body temperature is usually low, the pulse weak and rapid, and respirations shallow and possibly irregular. Deterioration in vital signs must be reported so that appropriate actions may be taken.

Neurological observations

Observation of the patient who suffers from trauma lesions or inflammatory processes of the nervous system is of vital importance to his well-being. Significant signs must be recognized and reported immediately so that appropriate and prompt action may prevent further damage which may be irreversible.

Head injuries

Injuries to the head may be open or closed. It is more likely with a closed injury that concussion and coma will occur because the skull is closed and there is increased pressure on the brain. Scalp wounds can be serious:
1 Because of bleeding.
2 A pathway for infection is made which may cause meningitis or abscesses.

Fractures of the skull

Any patient who has sustained an injury to the head must be examined for fractures and X-rayed.

Most fractures of the skull are simple and do not require treatment other than bed rest and observation of neurological signs. Complications which can occur as a result of simple fracture are haemorrhage of meningeal blood vessels with extradural or subdural haemorrhage, thrombosis leading to swelling of the brain, infection, meningitis or damage to nerves.

Depressed fractures of the skull need urgent treatment, so that intra cranial pressure can be relieved and bone fragments removed. Fractures of the base of the skull may involve the middle ear or paranasal sinuses. Vital centres in the medulla oblongata may be involved if the fracture is near the base of the skull.

Any individual who has severe scalp lacerations, fractures of the skull or loss of consciousness should be observed for at least 24 hours, as concussion, haemorrhage and intracranial compression may occur.

Concussion is characterized by loss of consciousness for a period which depends on the severity of the injury, the patient may be dazed when consciousness is regained.

Confusion may indicate more severe damage. There may have been small haemorrhages in the brain, causing weakness of limb or face and changes in speech. Evidence of cerebral irritation is shown by headache, and resentment when aroused. The individual turns away from the light and lies in a curled up position if he is undisturbed. The pulse usually exhibits a slow rate but a good volume, and the respiration is quiet and regular. Rising intracranial pressure may be caused by intracranial bleeding, or oedema of the brain. Unconsciousness will progressively deepen, and the pulse and respirations will slow down in rate and the blood pressure will rise. Immediate treatment is necessary.

Extradural haemorrhage may occur if the meningeal arteries are torn. Restlessness and headache may be the first signs, followed by dilatation of pupil on the affected side. The pulse rate usually slows and the respirations become stertorous, the blood pressure may rise and there is deepening unconsciousness. Immediate treatment is necessary to relieve the pressure.

On admission, the level of unconsciousness must be assessed and recorded accurately. The pupils are examined for size and reaction to light. The temperature, pulse, respiration and blood pressure are taken and recorded, together with signs that indicate changes in motor responses and sensory responses, i.e. is there obvious loss of power in limbs, is there normal reaction to pain, does the patient respond to speech, is his speech comprehensible or incomprehensible. Is there evidence of deafness, blindness, facial nerve palsy, a loss of cerebro spinal fluid through the nose or ears, or of neck rigidity? These observations and records provide a base line for comparison if the patient's condition deteriorates later.

Most trauma units have devised neurological observation charts on which the temperature, pulse, respiration, blood pressure, central venous pressure, pupil reaction, limb movements and coma scale are included with specific instructions for each section. The frequency of the recordings depends on the state of the patient and the severity of the injury. Often recordings are necessary at fifteen minute intervals and significant changes in temperature, pulse, respiration, blood pressure, level of consciousness, reaction of pupils, and motor and sensory responses must be recognized and reported immediately to the medical officer.

If the patient is sleeping or appears to be sleeping, he must be roused so that neurological observations can be made.

Nursing care required

This depends on the level of dependence of the patient. For the unconscious patient, positioning is of the utmost importance to:

a Keep the airway clear
b Prevent pressure
c Prevent inhalation of secretions
d Prevent injury to the limbs

Suction is of utmost importance to:

a Prevent inhalation of secretions
b Prevent hypostatic pneumonia
c If the cough reflex is absent or impaired, a tracheotomy may be performed for more efficient suction of the respiratory passages. Assisted respiration may be necessary.

Physiotherapy is of utmost import to:

a Prevent chest infections
b Prevent contraction of the limbs
c Prevent deep vein thrombosis

Fluids and nutrition to prevent dehydration and breakdown of tissues may be given by:

a Intravenous infusion
b Naso gastric feeding
c Fluid balance is recorded on an intake and output chart
d Where coma is prolonged, about 2000 calories are given daily through a naso gastric tube.

Medication

This is usually given by injection but may be given through the naso gastric tube. The patient's reaction to the medication has to be observed. Drugs may be used to reduce cerebral oedema, or anti-convulsants may be given if the patient has epileptic seizures due to injury. Narcotics are not usually given, e.g. morphine sulphate may mask signs of serious deterioration, or mimic serious signs, i.e. pinpoint pupils suggest injury to the brainstem, but may be caused by the admisistration of morphine sulphate.

Elimination

Quite often patients who have head injuries are incontinent of urine and steps have to be taken to keep the skin dry and clean to prevent soreness. However, restlessness in the unconscious patient may be due to retention of urine. To relieve this condition, an indwelling catheter may be passed and should be drained intermittently. Care has to be taken to prevent ascending infection when a patient has been catheterized. Constipation can be a problem for nursing the unconscious person, and this is usually relieved by giving evacuant suppositories to prevent impaction of faeces.

Eye care

While the patient is unconscious it is necessary to swab the eyelids to remove secretions and to irrigate the eyes with normal saline to prevent infection and damage to the cornea. Occasionally injuries to the brain prevent the eyelids closing normally, so it is necessary to instill sterile oils or ointment to prevent ulceration of the cornea. If pads are used to cover the eyes, make sure the eyelids are closed before the pads are applied.

The general hygiene of the patient must be attended to frequently and the mouth kept clean and moist and the hair neat. The area around the patient should not be cluttered. There should be enough space to work in wihout having to move equipment. Remember to talk to the patient while carrying out routine care and encourage the relatives to touch and talk to him.

If the patient has photophobia, prevent direct light from falling on his face. If the room is dark, changes in colour may not be seen.

Recovery of consciousness may be accompanied by restless movements, confusion and disorientation. The patient may get out of bed. The confusion may last for hours or days. Care has to be taken to prevent the patient from injury. Cot-sides may be used to try and keep him in bed. It is necessary that constant attention is given as in the recovery period patients may climb over cot-sides or slip out of the foot end of the bed causing further injury. If the patient is extremely restless, tranquilizers may be ordered. The effect has to be observed carefully. If there is no sign of restlessness abating, the medical staff should be informed. Observation of neurological signs is continued until the patient is showing signs of complete recovery.

Meningitis

This describes inflammation of the meninges which may be casued by bloodborn or airborn infection: influenzae virus, tubercle bacillus, streptococcus, staphylococcus and pneumococcus are usually the infecting organisms. The disease commonly occurs in children, but it may be as a result of direct infection from head injuries. Changes in vital signs that indicate meningitis are headache, vomiting, irritability to touch, photophobia, pyrexia and neck stiffness. There may be hyperpyrexia. Lumbar puncture is essential for diagnosis and appropriate antibiotics are given intravenously and systemically.

The response to treatment is monitored together with the vital signs. Signs of rising intracranial pressure in young children must be reported immediately. It may be necessary to perform a subdural tap to relieve the pressure.

Planning of nursing care depends on the level of dependence of the patient. It may be necessary to isolate the patient. General hygiene has to be attended to; frequent mouth washes or oral toilet are necessary as the mouth can be dry with fever. Attention must be paid to intake and output; if the patient is restless it may be due to a full bladder. For small children or the unconscious, fluids are usually given intravenously. Cooling procedures may be taken to reduce temperature and to make the patient as comfortable as possible.

Observations are made for response to drug therapy and for changes in neurological vital signs.

Practice Questions

Questions on vital signs

1 How is the constancy of body temperature maintained?
2 By what mechanism is body temperature controlled?
3 Describe the normal response of the vaso motor centre to increased body temperature.
4 Describe the normal response of the vaso motor centre to decreased body temperature.
5 What are pyrogens?
6 How do pyrogens affect the vaso motor centre?
7 State five major groups of conditions which cause fever.
8 What is the purpose of keeping neat and accurate temperature charts?
9 What are the commonly accepted variations in temperature in different parts of the body?
10 Give methods used to reduce body temperature.
11 Describe the characteristics of acute fever.
12 What does the term rigor describe?
13 Give the meaning of crisis and lysis.
14 Why do febrile convulsions occur in young children?
15 What general methods of nursing can be employed to ensure the comfort of the high dependence individual with fever?
16 In what circumstances is barrier nursing required?
17 When is it inadvisable to take body temperature by mouth?
18 What does hypothermia mean?
19 Who are people most at risk of hypothermia?
20 What reasons are there for inducing hypothermia?
21 Describe the events which occur if an individual suffers prolonged exposure.
22 Describe the main nursing responsibilities during and after the rewarming period.
23 Give the meanings of tachycardia and bradycardia.
24 Describe the origin and conduction of the heart beat.
25 What are the events in the cardiac cycle?
26 How is the nervous regulation of the heart mediated?
27 What may be the effects on heart action of:
   a   increase in potassium
   b   rise in PCO_2
   c   rise in blood pressure?
28 What does sinus rhythm mean?
29 What does arrhythmia describe?
30 What may cause tachycardia?
31 In which disease processes may tachycardia feature?
32 In which disease process may bradycardia be a feature?
33 What does extra systole describe?

34 What does paroxysmal tachycardia mean?
35 Describe the characteristics of the pulse due to atrial flutter.
36 Discuss the characteristics of the pulse in atrial fibrillation.
37 Why is it necessary to record apex and radial beats?
38 What do terms internal and external respiration mean?
39 How is respiration controlled?
40 What does dyspnoea mean?
41 What are the partial pressures of oxygen and carbon dioxide in arterial blood?
42 What are the partial pressures of oxygen and carbon dioxide in venous blood?
43 What are the reasons for using respiratory function tests?
44 What is the danger of using oxygen therapy in chronic respiratory disease?
45 Give reasons for Cheyne Stokes respirations.
46 What types of respirations are characteristically seen in pneumonia and acidosis?
47 What observations should be made whilst taking the respiratory rate?
48 What factors maintain blood pressure?
49 What do
  a hypertension and
  b hypotension mean respectively?
50 What does normotension mean?
51 What do systolic and diastolic pressure mean?
52 Give causes of hypertension.
53 What drugs are used in treatment of hypertension?
54 What are the signs of shock?
55 Define irreversible shock.
56 Describe the signs of concussion.
57 What complications may arise from simple head injury?
58 Describe signs of cerebral irritation.
59 What are the signs of rising intracranial pressure?
60 Describe how neurological vital signs are observed and the significant alterations in vital signs that should be reported.
61 What does vital capacity describe? Give the normal vital capacity for a healthy young man.

Answers to questions on vital signs
  1 Body temperature is maintained by heat loss and heat gain. In health, these processes are balanced and compensate for changes in temperature. Heat is lost by radiation, conduction, convection, evaporation, by water vapour from the respiratory tract, micturition and defaecation. Heat is gained by catabolic activity of cells, warmth and exercise.

2 Body temperature is controlled by:
  a The cerebral cortex, sensitive to changes in cutaneous temperature and responsible for initiating motor responses to deal with changes in temperature.
  b The vaso motor centre in the hypothalamus, which mediates its control via the autonomic nervous system and is sensitive to changes in cutaneous and blood temperature. This is the main centre.
3 The vaso motor centre reacts to a rise in body temperature in several ways:
  a It reduces impulses to peripheral blood vessels causing dilation, resulting in increased peripheral blood volume, so that heat loss by radiation, conduction and convection is increased.
  b There is increased stimulation of sweat glands so that heat is lost by evaporation of sweat.
  c There is reduced body activity of muscles and glands, thus less heat is produced.
  d There is voluntary relaxation and attempts to cool body or environment.
  Normal body temperature is usually restored by these efforts.
4 The vaso motor centre reacts to a drop in body temperature by:
  a Increasing impulses to peripheral blood vessels causing, constriction and resulting in reduced peripheral blood volume, so that heat loss by radiation, conduction, convection is reduced.
  b There is inhibition of sweat glands so that evaporation of heat by sweating is suppressed.
  c There is increased activity of muscles and glands, more heat is produced. Arector pili muscles in the skin help trap warmth.
  d There is voluntary activity and attempts to warm the body and environment.
  Body temperature is usually restored by these activities.
5 Pyrogens are substances thought to be released by leukocytes at the site of tissue damage.
6 The thermostat of the vaso motor centre is set at a higher level by the activity of pyrogens, consequently the normal reaction to a rise in body temperature does not occur until the concentration of pyrogens decreases.
7 Bacterial and viral infections, malignant disease, allergic conditions, systemic diseases, e.g. Crohn's disease or sarcoidosis, diseases of the brain or injury to the brain involving the vaso motor centre.
8 So that the pattern that fever takes may be clearly seen, this is an important aid to the diagnosis of fever, and to the condition of the patient.
9 Oral temperature ranges between 36°C-37°C. Usually, skin temper-

ature is about 0.5°C lower than oral temperature, rectal temperature is normally 1°C higher than oral temperature. If rectal temperature is taken, this should be marked on the chart.

10 By cooling the environment, giving fluids, cooling the body surface by cooling pads or tepid sponging. By administering drugs prescribed to reduce body temperature.

11 Shivering, headache, anorexia, rise in temperature and pulse rate, reduced urinary output, possibly rigor.

12 Usually characterises the onset of acute infections indicating pathogenic activity. The pattern is excessive shivering, during which the temperature rises steeply. When the new setting of the vaso motor centre is reached, the shivering stops and vasodilation occurs accompanied by sweating. The temperature returns to normal.

13 The term crisis describes a sudden change in an acute condition which may herald recovery or death. The term lysis describes a gradual return to normal temperature.

14 Febrile convulsions occur because the nervous system is not stabilised or completely developed.

15 Oral toilet, fluids, cooling measures, general hygiene, relief of constipation, help with moving, a quiet environment.

16 If the fever is of undetermined origin, it may be necessary to isolate an admission. Patients suffering from communicable diseases should be barrier nursed.

17 When the person is unconscious, unable to breathe through the nose, unable to take simple instructions, suffering from diseases in the mouth, or psychologically unreliable. It is not good practice to take oral temperatures when the individual is a child.

18 Lower than normal body temperature, placing the person at risk.

19 The elderly and small babies as they lose body heat more quickly than it is generated.

20 For therapeutic reasons, i.e. surgery or to treat hypertension and its damaging effects where brain damage has occurred.

21 The vaso motor centre is depressed, normal response to reduced body temperature does not occur. There is vasodilation, shivering stops, eventually the brain cells are damaged; there is confusion, sleep, coma, death.

22 Rewarming is a gradual process. The vital signs must be checked regularly, together with level of consciousness. The skin should be observed for discolouration and fluid intake and output recorded. It is necessary to observe the patient carefully for several days as arrhythmias may occur and there may be instability of heat controlling centres for some time.

23 Tachycardia describes a fast pulse rate. Bradycardia describes a slow pulse rate.

24 Impulses are discharged rhythmically from the sino-atrial node and spread as a wave of excitation through the muscles of the atria. The impulse is picked up by the atrioventicular node and is conducted to the venticular muscles by the bundle of His to the Purkinje system.

25 a Atrial systole 0.1 second
  b Ventricular systole 0.3 second
  c Relaxation of atria and ventricles 0.4 second.
  These events are known as the cardiac cycle.

26 By the cardiac inhibiting and accelerating centre in the medulla oblongata. Para sympathetic impulses slow down the rate of the heart, sympathetic impulses increase the heart rate.

27 a Causes abnormalities in conduction and convection, may lead to cardiac arrest.
  b Increase in heart rate over a period impairs conduction and contraction of heart rate.
  c Increase in blood pressure brings about a slowing in heart rate.

28 Regular heart action.

29 Irregular heart action.

30 Exercise, emotion, over-indulgence in coffee, alcohol or smoking.

31 Bleeding, fever, thyrotoxicosis.

32 Heart block, obstructive jaundice, raised intracranial pressure.

33 Irregular heart action.

34 Rapid impulses discharged from abnormal foci, which take over the function of the pace-maker, increasing the heart rate severely. The attacks may be of long or short duration.

35 Halving or doubling of pulse rate is characteristic of flutter.

36 The pulse is characteristically irregular in force and rhythm.

37 So that the difference between heart and pulse rate in conduction diseases can be noted, the general condition assessed and the response to treatment monitored.

38 External respiration is the process by which gases are interchanged between the air and the alveoli and the capillaries surrounding the alveoli. There is a constant exchange of oxygen and carbon dioxide between the individual and the environment. Internal respiration describes the process by which oxygen and nutrients are taken into the cells and waste products excreted.

39 By nervous and chemical control. The nerves in the respiratory centre are stimulated by sensory impulses and transient impulses to the spinal cord to initiate inspiration via the phrenic and intercostal nerves. Chemical control. Chemoreceptors are sensitive to oxygen lack and carbon dioxide excess. If PCO_2 rises and PO_2 decreases, the respirations increase.

40 Difficult and laborious respirations.

41 $PO_2 = 100$ mmHg. $PCO_2 = 38$ mmHg.

42 PO_2 = 40 mmHg. PCO_2 = 44 mmHg.

43 To estimate the respiratory ability of the individual.

44 Reduces the drive to the respiratory centre, so that respirations will be depressed.

45 The respiratory centre has a reduced sensitivity to PCO_2. Carbon dioxide is excreted by deep breathing, the respiratory centre is further depressed, the patient does not breathe for a short time, carbon dioxide builds up and the cycle starts again.

46 The respirations in lung infections are usually shallow and rapid; in acidosis breathing is deep.

47 The rate, character, depth, whether accessory muscles are used, whether the patient purses his lips on expiration, whether there are abnormal breath sounds. The colour of the patient should be observed, together with chest movements.

48 The force of the heart action and the output.
The volume and viscosity of blood in circulation.
The elasticity of arteries and the resistance of the peripheral arterioles.
Venous return.

49 a Means higher than normal blood pressure.
  b Means lower than normal blood pressure.

50 Blood pressure within normal limits for the individual.

51 The highest and lowest sounds heard in an artery as pressure is reduced in a sphygmomanometer cuff, correspond with systolic and diastolic blood pressure.

52 There are several causes of hypertension:
  a Essential hypertension may be due to increased peripheral resistance and decreased elasticity of arteries. 88% of people in this group.
  b Renal hypertension.
  c Hypertension associated with endocrine disease.
  d Hypertension associated with coarctation of the aorta.

53 Diuretics, sympathetic and ganglion blocking agents.

54 Pallor, sweating, air hunger, tachycardia, reduced pulse volume hypotension, vomiting, dimness of vision, fainting.

55 Irreversible shock occurs when compensatory mechanisms fail, causing damage to kidneys and brain cells.

56 Loss of consciousness with a dazed or disoriented behaviour when the patient recovers, there may be weakness of face or limbs and changes in speech.

57 Haemorrhage (internal or external), infection, thrombosis.

58 Headache, photophobia, resentment when touched, slow pulse of good volume.

59 Level of consciousness deteriorates, the pulse and respirations slow and the blood pressure rises.

60 Assess and record the level of consciousness, the temperature, pulse, respiratory rate and blood pressure. The size of the pupils and reaction to light are assessed, together with motor and sensory responses. Evidence of alteration in pupil reaction, deafness, blindness, facial or limb palsy, neck rigidity, loss of cerebro-spinal fluid must be reported, together with signs of deepening unconsciousness.

61 The sum of tidal volume, inspiratory reserve volume, expiratory reserve volume and residual volume. The vital capacity of a healthy young man is about 4.6 litres.

4 INVESTIGATIONS COMMONLY PERFORMED TO IDENTIFY DISEASE PROCESSES

The objectives of this section are to describe:
a The nurse's role in the investigation procedure.
b The reason for specific investigations.
c The interpretation of results.

Investigations cover a wide range of tests and procedures which may be carried out in the ward, laboratory, radiography department or operating theatre. The nurse's role in the investigation procedure is one of explanation and reassurance, of being able to identify the patient's needs and to deal with the patient's needs. It is essential that the patient is prepared for the tests following the instructions of the procedure committee, laboratory or radiography department. If tests have to be repeated because of inefficiency, there is increased anxiety for the patient and his family, and an increased strain on resources. When specimens are to be obtained on the ward, it is essential that instructions are followed carefully, that the patient is observed for reaction to the test or to drugs which may be administered. The specimens must be correctly labelled, i.e. dispatched to the laboratory with a correctly filled in card as soon as possible. The results should be read and interpreted and filed neatly in the patient's notes.

Tests on the urinary system and associated tests
First a brief recapitulation of the functions of the kidneys:
 i Maintenance of water and electrolytic balance.
 ii Maintenance of pH of body fluids.
 iii The excretion of end products of metabolism and drugs.
Second, the composition of urine:
 i 96% water.
 ii 4% solids: namely urea, uric acid, creatinine, chlorides, phosphates, potassium, calcium, magnesium, ammonia.
 iii pH is about 6.0 but varies with diet.
 iv The volume of urine in 24 hours is about 1.5 litres but this varies with intake of fluid, activity and temperature of the environment.
 v Specific gravity ranges between 1008–1025.
 vi Urochrome colours urine yellow, but occasionally foodstuffs and drugs alter the colour.

Investigation of urine
One of the first investigations performed in the out patient department or ward is a routine test of urine. A great deal of information can be obtained from this test, which may lead to further investigations. It is essential that abnormalities are quickly identified.

The principles of urine testing

1 Prevent infection. The urine testing area should be clean and surfaces dry. Hands should be clean and the uniform protected.

2 The agents for urine testing should be stored and used according to manufacturer's instructions; damp or exposed agents will deteriorate.

3 The urine should be collected in a clean container. If it is not to be tested immediately it should be covered and labelled with time and date of collection, and the patient's name.

4 Points to be noted for urine testing.

   a Observe colour and sediment, note the volume and specific gravity. The specific gravity gives information about the kidney's ability to concentrate and dilute; it will be higher than normal if abnormal constituents are present. e.g. sugar. Normal specific gravity ranges between 1008—1025. If the volume of urine obtained is inadequate to test specific gravity a narrow container can be used so that the urinometer will float and record specific gravity accurately. Note the odour of urine. Urine has a characteristic smell; significant odours are fishy or sweet smells.

   b Reaction of urine is normally acid pH6, but it may be alkaline. Reaction should always be noted.

   c Routine urine test may be performed with labstix, or it may be necessary to carry out tests separately for protein, bile, blood, ketones or glucose. Chemical analysis may be required.

Indiviual tests

Tests for sugar comprises Clinistix, Clinitest tablets or Benedicts test. Reagents must be stores carefully according to manufacturers's instructions or false positive results may be obtained. Glycosuria does not necessarily indicate the presence of diabetes mellitus. Medication with salicylates may produce a positive clinitest reaction many young people have renal glycosuria without a raised blood sugar. Sugar may be seen in the urine after partial Gastrectomy, and in the urine of about 25% of pregnant women. If it is thought to be a significant finding other tests such as blood sugar estimation and glucose tolerance tests may be carried out.

Tests of ketones

The Rothera Test and Acetest tablets are tests for Acetone. The normal person excretes about 100 mgm of ketones daily. Ketosis occurs in a wide variety of illnesses such as starvation (crash dieting), myocardial infarction, pneumonia. In diabetic ketosis the normal amount of ketones excreted daily is excessive; any significant change in the urine of a patient with diabetes must be noted and reported. It should be noted that patients treated with phenformin may have ketonuria.

Test for protein

A small amount of protein may be found in the urine of healthy individuals.

The types of test available to test urine for albumen or protein include the Albustix test which is commonly used. Occasionally the boiling test may be asked for if there is sediment in the urine, or if an Albustix test is positive. Acidification of urine after boiling dissolves inorganic phosphates, but does not dissolve coagulated protein. If significant amounts of protein are found in the urine, tests on blood and more sophisticated tests on urine will be carried out.

Blood in urine

The test used is the Ames tablet test. Always ascertain whether a lady patient is menstruating prior to collecting urine; if this is the case make sure the genitalia are clean and the vagina is plugged before collecting the specimen. Other than this blood in the urine may arise from disease or injury in the renal tract, or it may result from treatment with anticoagulents. Blood in the urine may be obvious, it may alter the colour of the urine, or it may be almost undetectable. Positive reaction to the test should be reported.

Bile in the urine

Bilirubin in the urine is present in cases of obstructive jaundice. It alters the colour of the urine significantly to a green or brown colour. The test carried out is the Ames test.

All the Ames tests should be carried out according to the manufacturer's instructions. All the reagents must be stored carefully and must not be allowed to come into contact with water or be stored in damp areas.

Notes on urine tests must be made immediately; if charts are used, clear and accurate recordings should be made. For four hourly tests of urine of diabetic patients, significant changes in sugar + ketone content must be reported.

Mid-stream collections of urine

Follow the instructions laid down in the procedure book. Make sure the patient understands the procedure and that the external genitalia are clean. The principle involved is to collect the middle of the flow of urine. The first portion of urine passed is discarded as it will contain bacteria from inside the urethra. The middle flow of urine is collected in a sterile container and then transferred to a universal container which is correctly labelled and sent to the laboratory, along with a request card signed by the doctor. If the urine is not collected carefully a false positive result can be obtained.

A clean catch specimen means that the whole specimen of urine is collected in a clean container, after the genitalia have been washed. The specimen is put into a jar, labelled and sent to the laboratory with a request card.

The 24 hour collection of urine
The 24 hour collection of urine may be requested for many reasons. The rules of the procedure book should be followed, but **all** urine passed in 24 hours should be collected. The correct container for the required test must be obtained from the laboratory and labelled with the patient's name. The specific gravity and reaction of each specimen should be tested and recorded, together with the volume of urine passed. A qualitative estimate of, e.g. protein, hormones, glucose or electrolytes can be obtained from a 24 hour urine collection.

Investigation of the respiratory tract
One of the first investigations will be made by the admitting nurse who takes and records the vital signs (see chapter dealing with vital signs). Relevant information is obtained with regard to the patient's respiratory ability, his general well-being and normal functions. His needs are identified and dealt with if possible.
Signs of respiratory disease are cough, alteration in rate, rhythm and volume of respirations, changes in respiratory excursions, pain, alteration in breath sounds and chest movements, and cyanosis.
Investigation is necessary to identify the disease process or organism that may be the cause of the problem.

Investigation of cardiovascular system
One of the first investigations of the cardiovascular system is made by the admitting nurse who interviews the patient, observes his physical ability and notes his colour and vital signs.

Test commonly carried out to investigate heart disease
Pulse, respiration and blood pressure recordings are taken. Alterations from normal may be significant of disease. (See chapter dealing with vital signs.)
A chest X-ray is done to assess the size and shape of the heart, aorta and pulmonary artery. Density of the lungs may show fluid or back-flow of blood in the lungs.

Electrocardiography
This is a test to measure the electrical impulses generated from heart activity as they reach the body surface. Electrodes and jelly are applied to specific areas of the body. These are attached to the electrocardiogram. Impulses are recorded at specific areas and recorded on graph paper by

Disease	Volume in 24 hrs	Specific gravity	Appearance
Diabetes mellitus (uncontrolled)	Increased	Increased	Pale
Pyelitis and cystitis	Often decreased	No change usually	Cloudy mucus Ammonia smell
Tubercle of kidney or bladder	N.S.C. (No significant change)	N.S.C.	May be bloodstained
Renal or bladder calculi	N.S.C.	N.S.C.	May be bloodstained
Acute glomerular nephritis	Decreased	High	Smokey from blood cells
Nephrotic syndrome	Normal	No change initially, low later	Pale
Acute renal failure	Reduced↓ Oliguria↓ Anuria	May be raised	Concentrated
Essential hypertension	May be increased	Normal or low	N.S.C.
Chronic renal failure	Increased	Low and fixed	Pale
Obstructive jaundice		May be increased	Dark brown or green

found on ward examination of urine

Protein	Blood	Ketones	Sugar	Bile	Deposits	Further investigation that may be ordered
		+ ve	+ ve			24 hr urine collection m.s.u. blood sugar Glucose tolerance tests
+ ve	+ ve				Pus bacteria	m.s.u. + microscopy
					Pus tubercle bacillus	m.s.u. Urine for 24 hr collection and Tubercle bacilicus 3 consecutive early morning specimens. X-Rays of renal tract and lungs are collected.
+ ve	+ ve				Bacteria	Blood urea. m.s.u, i.v.p. Cytoscopy. Retrograde pyelography. 24 hr urine collection.
+ ve	+ ve				Red cells + casts	Blood urea. 24 hr urine collection. Daily protein estimation and electrolytes E.S.R.
Large amounts					Casts + possibly red cells	Blood urea and electrolytes with plasma proteins; i.v.p. Renal function tests. 24 hour urine collections. Renal biopsy.
						Blood urea. Electrolytes. Serum proteins, E.C.G. Haemoglobin.
+ ve					Casts	Blood urea. Electrolytes. i.v.p, urine tests,. E.C.G. Angiography
+ ve in small amounts					Casts + red cells	Blood urea. Electrolytes Plasma proteins. 24 hr urine collections. Renal function tests
				+ ve		Liver function tests Cholecystography

Examples of tests carried out on the renal tract apart from ward routine

Tests	Specimens or preparation required	Reason for tests
Blood chemistry	Venous blood	Damage to glomeruli or tubules causes change in blood urea, S Albumen, S Calcium, S Sodium and S Potassium.
Creatinine clearance	10 ml of venous blood 24 hour collection of urine.	To estimate the rate of clearance through the glomeruli.
Concentration and dilution test	2 tests involved on urine **1st.** 3 specimens of urine from a fasting patient. **2nd.** in 24 hours. A larger fluid intake is given and four specimens of urine are collected in four hours.	Tests the ability of the kidneys to deal with fluid restriction, followed by a test of the kidneys to deal with a high intake of fluid.
Intravenous pyelography	Explanation of test. Identify allergies. Empty bowel to evacuate gas. Fast for 12 hrs. Watch for reaction to hypaque.	To examine the structure and function of the urinary tract by injecting a radiopaque substance intravenously. X-Rays are taken at 5, 10 and 20 mins.
Cystoscopy	Explanation of test. Consent obtained. Evacuation of bowel, general preparation for G.A. or L.A.	To examine the interior of the bladder and ureteric orifices via a lighted tube (a cystoscope).
Retrograde pyelogram	Usually done under L.A. Explanation and consent necessary. After procedure is completed, measure urine passed and observe amount of haematuria — a rise in temperature should be reported.	To pass ureteric catheters into both ureters, so that urine may be collected and dye injected.
Renal angiography	Explanation. Consent for test under L.A.	The technique is similar to i.v.p. Renal vessels are examined.
Renal biopsy	Explanation. Consent. Prepare trolley, place patient in prone position. Keep patient in bed for 24 hours after. Observe and report backache, haematuria and urinary output.	To obtain a piece of kidney tissue for examination.

tests & m.s.u.

Normal values or reactions	Results
Blood urea 3-7 mmol/litre S Albumen 3.5 . 5.5 mEq/litre S Calcium 4.5 . 6.0 mEq/litre S Sodium 135-145 mmol/litre S Potassium 3.6 . 5.0 mmol/litre	— Raised in impactment — decreased in kidney disease — low in chronic nephritis — low in chronic renal failure — low in chronic renal failure
70-130/ml per minute clearance rate.	Rate is decreased in disease and may be 5/ml per minute.
For the 1st test on 3 specimens the specific gravity should not fall below 1024. For the 2nd test the specific gravity should rise above 1002.	Fixed specific gravity at 1010 during both tests indicates renal damage.
The normal kidney will excrete dye and make the tract opaque to X-ray.	If the kidneys are diseased the dye will not be excreted. Stones and abnormalities may be seen.
Normally the bladder wall and orifices are clearly defined.	Abnormalities such as stones or casts may be seen. Abnormalities such as stones and growths may be seen in ureters, pelvis and kidney.
	Structures or abnormalities of blood vessels may be identified.
	Will identify disease which is difficult to diagnose by other means.

Tests	Reason for investigation	Specimens required
Plain chest X-ray	To ascertain visual information about the state of the lungs.	—
Bronchography	To examine the state of the bronchial tree using contrast media.	—
Bacteriological tests and cytology tests	To isolate organisms causing disease or to identify pathological processes. Smears or cultures may be done.	Sputum
Bacteriological tests and cyctology tests	To identify causes of pleural effusion.	Pleural fluid

(continued on following page)

the respiratory tract

Care of patients undergoing investigations	Results
Explain the X-ray procedure Explain the reason for the X-ray. Postural drainage may be required beforehand. Prepare patient for X-ray. Postural drainage may be necessary on completion of procedure to drain out contrast media.	May show extent of tissue damage, or outline lesions. May show the extent of involvement in disease process of the bronchial tree.
Explain the procedure. Sputum is collected in the early morning so that a higher concentration of bacteria may be present. The patient is instructed to expectorate into a container, once obtained the specimen is covered labelled and sent to the laboratory within two hours. Occasionally 3 consecutive early morning specimens may be required.	Bacteria causing chest infection may be identified i.e. pneumococcus, streptococcus, influenzae, malignant cells or tubercle. Casts may be seen in the sputum of asthmatic patients.
Explain the procedure to the patient and obtain consent. Obtain X-rays. Prepare for pleural tap according to procedure committee instructions. Record vital signs during tap, make sure the puncture is sealed.	Bacteria e.g. pneumococcus or tubercle may be identified.

Tests	Reason for investigation	Specimens required
Bacteriological tests and cytology tests.	To ascertain pleural tissue to identify cause of disease. Usually done when diagnosis is difficult.	Pleural tissue
Endoscopic examination	To examine the respiratory tract under direct vision.	Tissue
Laryngoscopy	To remove foreign bodies i.e. mucous plugs, or tissue for histological examination.	Tissue
Bronchoscopy	To remove tissue for histological examination.	Tissue
Bronchial washing may be done	To examine cells from the bronchi.	

Refer to section on vital signs for tests on blood and for respiratory function tests.

Care of patients undergoing Investigation	Results
Record vital signs for 4 hours after tap, note alterations in colour i.e. greyness or cyanosis. Report alterations in respiratory rate and observe whether both sides of the chest are moving. Note and deal with complaints of pain.	
As for pleural tap excepting for a small incision which will be sutured. The suture will have to be removed in 3-4 days.	Bacteria or tubercle or malignant cells may be identified.
Explain the reason for the examination. Obtain previous X-rays. Obtain consent for G.A. When the procedure is complete the patient is cared for until conscious as for any post operative patient. Observe vital signs, especially colour, respiration, alteration in breath sounds. The patient may complain of hoarseness or sore throat after this examination.	Malignant disease may be identified. A direct visual inspection provides more detailed information to the surgeon as to the state and function of the respiratory tract. Malignant cells may be identified.

the electrocardiograph. The waves are called P.Q.R.S.T. waves. The P wave represents activity of the atria, the Q.R.S. waves transmission of impulses from the atria to the ventricles. The time lapse between conduction from the atria to the ventricles is demonstrated by the PR interval. The T wave co-relates with the recovery of the ventricular muscle. The tracing is read immediately; comparisons are made with tracings of a healthy heart. Information can be gained about the initiation of impulses, strength of conduction, the state of the ventricles and the response of the heart to impulses. Drugs may alter the heart action and a note should be made on the graph if drugs such as Digoxin are being taken. The patient is watched carefully during the procedure for any abnormal reactions. Remember to clean the skin when the electrodes are removed.

For tests of vital capacity — See chapter on vital signs.

Angiography
This test is done to view the heart and blood vessels, and is of importance in identifying diseased or damaged vessels and congenital heart defects. A radio opaque fluid is inserted and X-rays are taken. Cine-radiography is also carried out.
The patient fasts, consent must be obtained for the procedure and allergies are identified. Observation when the test is complete involves vital signs and examination for thrombosis.

Cardiac catheterization
This is performed:
a To detect congenital defects.
b To determine blood pressure in atria and ventricles.
c To obtain specimens of blood to estimate PO_2 in various chambers of the heart.

Principle
The procedure is explained and consent obtained for the examination. The examination may be conducted under general or local anaesthetic. Cardiac catheters are passed under the guidance of fluoroscopes. The left and right side of the heart are examined separately. Radio opaque fluids are injected and X-rays are taken.
After the procedure is completed, observation of vital signs is made. If the pulse becomes weak or irregular, the doctor should be informed. The site of injection of the catheter should be inspected for irritation or thrombosis. For right-sided catheterization, the basilic vein in the right arm may be used; for left-sided catheterization a femoral artery is used. Blood tests done in cardiac disease depend on the patient's signs and symptoms.

Generally, a full blood count is done to estimate:

a The numbers of erythrocytes, size, shape and haemoglobin content.

b White cell count and differential count.

c Platelet count.

Erythrocyte sedimentation rate, if raised, gives an indication of inflammatory activity, e.g. ESR is raised in myocardial infarction.

Measurements of blood gas tensions help in evaluating the cause of cyanosis.

Measurement of heart muscle enzymes released into the blood during infarction and after infarction give a guide to the severity of damage. S.G.O.T. rises quickly after infarction and returns to normal in about a week. S.L.D.H. rises more slowly and returns to normal in about 10 days.

Blood culture specimens are taken to identify the organism present in subacute bacterial endocarditis. Usually streptococcus viridans is present, though streptococcus faecalis may be found.

Investigation of the alimentary tract

The type of tests performed will depend on the underlying disease process and include studies of blood, gastric and intestinal juices, stools and urine, together with endoscopy and barium studies.

History

Information should be obtained on admission regarding appetite, ability to eat any food, difficulty in swallowing, change in bowel habit, in colour of skin, urine or faeces. The vital signs should be taken and recorded and used as a baseline. Pain, changes in colour, stools, urine or passing of blood in stools or vomit are significant and should be reported.

Blood in vomit or haematemesis

The volume and frequency of blood in vomit should be noted. Blood in vomit may be due to swallowing blood, or coughing up blood, but usually haematemesis is dark, acid and there may be clots of blood.

Blood in faeces

This may be due to haemorrhoids, new growths or fissures, Crohn's disease or ulcerative colitis. Melaena, which indicates bleeding from high in the gastro intestinal tract, may be slight or have a characteristically black and tarry appearance. If the patient is bleeding, the vital signs should be checked frequently. Any change in bowel habit should be reported.

Patients who are to undergo tests of the alimentary tract should be given an explanation and consent should be obtained for the procedure.

Endoscopy

This involves visual examination by a lighted instrument called an endoscope. Preparation depends on the examination, i.e. proctoscopy is done in the ward without special preparation. Examinations of stomach, duodenum, small and large intestine involve preparation according to the instructions of the doctor concerned. Steps are taken to ensure the stomach and bowel are clear of solids. The tests may be performed under general anaesthetic in some cases.

Examples of tests are;

Oesophagoscopy — an examination of the oesophagus.

Gastroscopy and fibroscopy — an examination of the stomach.

Duodenoscopy and examination of the duodenum.

Sigmoidoscopy — an examination of the colon.

Barium studies involve radiological examination of the gastro intestinal tract. Preparation involves fasting overnight and emptying the stomach and bowel of solids. For upper gastro intestinal tests, the patient is asked to swallow barium sulphate. For lower bowel studies, barium is introduced with a catheter i.e. barium enema. The gastro intestinal tract is screened and X-rays are taken. Barium sulphate is a non-toxic radio opaque substance. Occasionally, patients need laxatives after barium swallow and barium meal to evacuate barium from the bowel.

Gastric function tests are performed to:

1 Assess the reaction of the stomach to a stimulant.
2 Measure the night juice secretions.
3 Assess the efficiency of vagotamy.

In most cases, a naso gastric tube is passed to obtain specimens. Very occasionally, the tubeless test meal is used. The tests are conducted according to instructions and the patient should be observed for adverse reactions if gastric stimulants are used.

Stool examination

The type of preparation the patient is required to undergo depends on the reason for the investigation, i.e. stools may be tested for blood using the haematest tablet method in the ward, requiring no specific preparation. If hidden blood loss is suspected, usually a three-day collection of faeces for occult blood is made. For fat tests, the whole of the stool is collected. A fresh specimen of stool is sent to the laboratory immediately if parasitic infection is suspected.

Other tests necessary to complete the investigation

A full blood picture is taken together with plain chest and abdominal x-rays.

For diseases of the oesophagus
Barium swallow is carried out which may identify lesions and their position. Oesophagoscopy involves a visual examination to be made. During the examination, foreign bodies may be removed, or strictures may be dilated and specimens of tissue taken for histological examination. Vital signs should be checked carefully after the examination, as there is a risk of mediastinitis. Blood will be taken for full blood count.

For diseases of the stomach
Barium meal is carried out which may demonstrate filling defects, indicating the size and position of lesions in the stomach. Gastroscopy or fibroscopy enable a visual examination to be made of the interior of the stomach. Photographs of significant areas may be taken, together with tissue for histological examination. Patients may experience sore throats or flatulence after this examination. The result of gastric function tests may show achlorhydria if there is atrophy of gastric mucosa as in pernicious anaemia or carcinoma. Hyperchlorhydria is associated with duodenal ulcer. Raised resting juice and residual fluid are associated with slow emptying of the stomach. Blood will be taken for full blood count.

For diseases of the duodenum
Duodenoscopy may be performed to examine the inside of the duodenum and to obtain tissue for examination. Barium meal and follow through may outline deformities of the duodenal cap associated with duodenal ulcer. Gastric function test shows a rise in H.C.L. Stools collection for occult blood may also be required. Blood will be taken for full blood count.

For diseases of the large intestine
Barium enema is necessary, together with sigmoidoscopy and tissue biopsy. Tissue biopsy may show inflammatory changes or malignant disease. Barium studies identify the site and outline of structures or filling defects.

For diseases of the small and large intestine, i.e. Crohn's disease or ulcerative colitis
Barium meal and follow through, and barium enema are necessary to identify lesions. Stools collection for occult blood and faecal fat are necessary. A full blood picture is necessary.

For diseases of the gall bladder and biliary tract
Blood tests called liver function tests will be done. In obstructive jaundice, the serum bilirubin is raised. S.G.O.T. may be slightly raised;

serum alkaline phosphatase is usually raised. Urine and stools are observed for changes in colour, i.e. in obstructive jaundice bile is present in urine and absent from stools. Barium meal is usually carried out and examination of the gall bladder and bile ducts e.g. cholecystography and cholangiography.

For acute and chronic pancreatitis

It is necessary to collect stools to estimate faecal fat. The level of serum amylase in the blood will be raised and the level of excretion of urinary amylase. Specimens needed: venous blood, faeces and 24 hour urine collection.

The preparation guide lines for the above investigations must be followed correctly or patients may have to undergo unnecessary repeat investigations. The results of the test and investigations should be obtained from the appropriate departments and filed in the patient's notes. X-rays should be ready with the radiologist's report for the surgeon to scrutinise as soon as possible.

The patient and his relatives should be informed of the findings as soon as possible so that unnecessary worry may be relieved.

Neurological tests

Neurological tests may be done in wards or departments. The responsibility of the nurse lies in preparation of the patient and equipment for the tests.

The neurological trolley should be prepared according to the instructions of the procedure book.

It may be necessary to interview relatives before or after the examination as they may be able to describe significant changes in the patient's appearance or behaviour.

During a physical examination of the patient, the size, shape and strength of muscles will be assessed, together with the ability to move easily in a coordinated manner and to carry out simple requests to pick up or identify objects with the eyes closed. The size of limbs, length and girth are measured and wasting is noted. Any spasticity, flaccidity or paralysis of muscles is noted, as these are common signs of neurological disturbance.

Upper motor neurone lesions produce spasticity of muscles, lower motor neurone lesions produce flaccidity of muscles. Fine tremor may be seen as a result of anxiety, tension, drugs or overactivity of the thyroid gland. Intention tremor is seen in patients who have Parkinson's disease. Movements are very exaggerated when trying to reach an object: this is due to degeneration of the basal ganglia. A tic may be associated with habit or nervousness. There may be local convulsive movements of one part of the body or generalised convulsions. Incoordination or inability of groups of muscles to perform certain acts is seen in diseases of the central nervous system, e.g. cerebral tumour, multiple sclerosis. There may be abnormality of gait. The person with Parkinson's disease has a characteristic shuffle and there may be staggering or erratic movements characteristic of diseases in the cerebellum.

Reflex actions are tested using a tendon hammer. Superficial reflexes are examined by stroking the skin (i.e. the skin of the abdomen is stroked, contraction of muscles should be the reaction), and deep reflexes by striking the tendon. Normal reaction to the maxillary reflex is closure of jaw, to the biceps tendon flexion of the elbow, to the triceps tendon flexion of the forearm, to the patella tendon contraction of quadriceps and extension of leg, to the achilles tendon calf muscles contract, and to plantar stimulation flexion of the toes.

Babinski's sign is normally present up to two years of age. After two years of age, the sign is significant of disease involving upper motor neurones.

In diseases of the central nervous system, the response to reflex stimulation may be exaggerated or absent, i.e. the knee jerk is absent in lower motor neurone disease and increased in upper motor neurone disease.

The normal response to corneal stimulation should be closing of eyelid, to pupil stimulation contraction to light, and to accommodation should be contraction of pupil when focusing on a near object after looking at a distant object.

Interference with pathways of sensation may result in increased or decreased sensitivity to touch, temperature, pain. The reaction to tests will give valuable information regarding underlying lesions. The patient may be unable to distinguish between painful stimulation and stroking, or be unable to recognize heat or cold on an area. The ability to feel vibrations when a tuning fork is placed on the body surface is tested and also the ability to recognize objects placed in the hand while the eyes are closed.

It may be necessary to test various cranial nerves when there are injuries to or diseases of the central nervous system.

Cranial nerve I is tested with aromatic odours. The ability to identify or recognize differences in odours is important. In head injuries involving the olfactory nerve, the senses of smell and taste are inhibited.

Cranial nerve II Vision is tested for ability, colour and perimetry. In lesions of the brain, fields of vision may be significantly affected, with loss of half, or all of vision. The optic nerves can be examined directly with an ophthalmoscope.

Cranial nerves III, IV and VI are responsible for movements of eyeballs and eyelids. If there is damage, there may be alteration in movement of the eyeball, squint or double vision or ptosis of eyelid.

Cranial nerve V The trigeminal nerve may be damaged as a result of shingles or neuralgia, with hypersensitivity of scalp and loss of sensation in the cornea. In acute stages, it may be necessary to shield the eye to prevent corneal ulceration.

Cranial nerve VII The facial nerve supplies the muscles of the face. If paralysed, there is difficulty in closing the eye, the face is not symmetrical and the lips do not purse easily.

Cranial nerve VIII The auditory nerve supplies the inner ear and the semicircular canals. Deafness may occur as a result of loss of conduction of sound due to disease in the middle ear, or the nerve may be damaged; the individual will not be able to perceive sound. An auroscope may be used to examine the auditory canal and typanic membrane. Audiometry tests are carried out to estimate the level of hearing. Symptoms of disturbance in the semicircular canals are dizziness, loss of balance and vomiting and nystagmus. Water tests called the caloric tests are used to estimate the degree of disturbance in balance.

Cranial nerves IX Glossopharyngeal, **X** Vagus, **XI** Accessory, and **XII** Hypoglossal. These may all be involved in the same lesion, though lesions may occur individually and there may be dysphagia or paralysis of the recurrent laryngeal nerve, dropping shoulder or weakness of the tongue. Examinations carried out to diagnose diseases of the nervous system are blood tests, electro-encephalogram to assess brain activity, lumbar puncture and cisternal puncture to examine the cerebrospinal fluid. Other test include arteriogram, encephalogram, ventriculogram, myelogram.

Tests for meningeal irritation are:
1 Neck rigidity — Normally the neck flexes quite far onto the chest but flexion is limited in meningeal irritation and there is pain.
2 Kernig's sign — Normally the thigh, when flexed, will straighten easily. However, if the thigh is flexed when meningeal irritation is present, it will not straighten easily, the muscles contract and pain is experienced.
1 and **2** are positive signs of meningeal irritation.

Blood investigation procedures for common blood disorders
Tests usually carried out to investigate blood disorders are performed on venous blood, on bone marrow specimens, on gastric juice, stools and urine. In certain cases it may be necessary to take a biopsy of an involved lymph node for histology.

Test on blood to diagnose erythrocyte disorders
These include E.S.R., red blood cell count, haemoglobin content of erythrocytes, packed cell volume and erythrocytic indices. Reticulocytic

count and fragility tests may be necessary. In red blood cell disorders certain changes occur in the cells. Erythrocytes that are larger than normal are described as macrocytic, those smaller than normal are described as microcytic. Cells with a deficiency of haemoglobin are called normochromic, cells with an excess of haemoglobin are called hypochromic cells with an excess of haemoglobin are called hyperchromic. Anaemias are usually classified according to the changes in the cells i.e. microcytic hyperchromic cells are usually seen in iron deficiency anaemias, macrocytic hyperchromic cells are usually seen in vitamin B_{12} anaemias. The erythrocyte sedimentation rate in anaemia is usually raised and packed cell volume is usually reduced.

White cell disorders
White cells are counted at the same time as the red cells. An increase in white cells known as leucocytosis occurs as a result of infections e.g. pneumonia or appendicitis. Leucopenia means a decrease in white cells, and occurs as a result of drugs, poisons, irradiation, aplastic anaemia and typhoid fever. A great increase in white cells occurs in most types of leukaemia and abnormal cells are seen. The function of platelets is to take part in the process of clotting. Platelets are reduced in aplastic anaemia, acute leukaemia, and auto immune disease. The platelet count is usually increased after splenectomy. Only examples of tests are included here. Any patient undergoing investigation will be anxious, therefore the reason for the test should be explained. It may be necessary to observe the puncture site after blood has been taken for bleeding or bruising; if a dressing is applied make sure the patient is not allergic to adhesive tape.

Normal values of blood

White cells	4–11×10^9/litre.
Erythrocytes	4–6×10^{12}/litre.
Platelets	150–400×10^9/litre.
Bleeding time	1–6 minutes.
Clotting time	4–10 minutes.
Haemoglobin	12–18 g/dl
pH	7.35–7.45
pCO_2	5.6 kPa
pO_2	11–15 kPa

Bone marrow puncture
Examination of the bone marrow is important in diagnosis of blood disorders. The sites for puncture usually chosen are the sternum and iliac crest. The procedure is explained, the patient is prepared and local anaesthetic is given. The bone marrow is punctured with a marrow puncture trocar and cannula, the trocar is removed and marrow is sucked

out with a syringe. The marrow is spread immediately on to slides and taken to the laboratory. The puncture wound is covered. The number of cells are counted and the various stages of development are observed; the size, shape and characteristics of the cells are noted. This procedure confirms pernicious anaemia, leukaemia and other blood disorders.

Gastric function tests

The secretion of gastric juice varies in different people, and there are variations in different diseases. Impaired absorption of iron may result from achlorhydria, after gastrectomy or from malabsorption in the intestine. In pernicious anaemia the intrinsic factor is absent, therefore B_{12} cannot be naturally absorbed. Therefore it may be necessary to investigate the contents of gastric juice and the reaction of the stomach to a stimulant. Tests commonly used are **a** the augmented histamine test **b** the pentagastrin test and **c** the Schilling test. For **a** and **b** a nasogastric tube is passed. A stimulant is given and the test is carried out according to the procedure rules. For **c** radioactive B_{12} is given orally to a fasting patient. A large dose of B_{12} is given intramuscularly and a gastric stimulant is given. All urine is collected for 24 hours. Normally 7% of the radioactive dose is excreted. This is considerably reduced in pernicious anaemia; if a small amount is excreted this test is followed by a second test. Intrinsic factor is usually given if the amount excreted is normal; pernicious anaemia is usually diagnosed. Less than normal excreted indicates intestinal malabsorption.

Urinary urobilinogen

The urobilinogen excreted in urine is estimated,
normal = 0 to 4 mgm in 24 hours. It is increased in excessive red cell destruction and in liver disease.

Faceal urobilinogen

The urobilinogen excreted in faeces is estimated,
normal = 50–300 mgm in 24 hours. It is increased in excessive red cell destruction.

Occult blood test

Stools may be tested for hidden blood as part of the investigation. See tests on the alimentary tract.

Practice Questions

Questions on investigations

 1 State the functions of the kidneys.
 2 Give the normal constituents of urine.
 3 Why is urine tested?
 4 What abnormalities may be found in urine that do not indicate disease?
 5 What is the significance of sugar and ketones in the urine?
 6 Why are mid-stream specimens of urine taken?
 7 Give the meaning of oliguria, anuria, suppression of urine, polydipsia, polyuria.
 8 For what reasons are 24 hour collections of urine made?
 9 What is the normal level of blood urea?
 10 What is the significance of raised blood urea?
 11 What is the significance of fixed low specific gravity in urine?
 12 What are the features of nephrotic syndrome?
 13 What does haematuria mean?
 14 Give the causes of blood in the urine.
 15 State the significance of bile in the urine.
 16 What further tests are necessary if bile is found in the urine?
 17 Why is intravenous pyelography performed in relation to investigation of the urinary system?
 18 For what reason is cystoscopy performed?
 19 Why is intravenous pyelography performed in relation to tests on the renal tract?
 20 For what reason is renal angiography performed?
 21 Why is renal biopsy performed?
 22 State the dangers of injecting hypaque for X-ray examinations.
 23 Give the care necessary following:
    a   retrograde pyelography
    b   intravenous pyelography
    c   renal biopsy
 24 What are the signs of urinary tract infection?
 25 Why are a bronchoscopy and b bronchography performed?
 26 What information may be obtained from analysis of sputum?
 27 What methods can be used to relieve pain and congestion in the lungs?
 28 State the observations necessary after pleural tap and biopsy.
 29 What information can be obtained from E.C.G. recordings?
 30 What is the significance of raised erythrocyte sedimentation rate?
 31 State the observations necessary after cardiac catheterization.
 32 What may be the causative organism of bacterial endocarditis?
 33 What is the significance of S.G.O.T. and S. L.D.H. in blood?
 34 Define anaemia.

35 Give the normal numbers of erythrocytes in blood.
36 What are the changes in cells in **a** iron deficiency anaemia and **b** pernicious anaemia?
37 What does aplastic anaemia mean?
38 What investigations are carried out to identify types of anaemia?
39 What does achlorhydria mean?
40 In what condition may hyperchlorhydria occur?
41 What do the terms **a** melaena and **b** haematemesis mean?
42 What does endoscopy mean?
43 State the endoscopic examinations done to examine the gastro intestinal tract.
44 Name the barium studies necessary to investigate the gastro intestinal tract.
45 What does occult blood mean?
46 What does Babinski's sign indicate?
47 What does Kernig's sign indicate?
48 What examinations are carried out to investigate diseases of the nervous system?
49 What are the signs of meningitis?
50 Give the normal numbers of white blood cells in circulation.
51 What does leucocytosis indicate?
52 What does leucopenia mean?
53 Give the normal numbers of platelets in circulation.
54 What does hyperchlorhydria mean?

Answers to questions on investigations

1 Maintenance of water and electrolytic balance. Maintenance of pH of body fluids. Excretion of end products of metabolism and drugs.
2 96% water, 4% solids = urea, uric acid, creatinine, chlorides, phosphates, potassium, calcium, magnesium, ammonia.
3 To obtain baseline information about the efficiency of the kidney and to identify abnormalities that may indicate underlying disease which will need further investigation.
4 Protein in urine may not be an abnormality, but may result from back pressure on the kidneys, i.e. soldiers on parade for many hours have incidence of protein in urine. Glucose may indicate high carbohydrate intake, lactose is present in the urine of lactacting women, Salicylates may bring about a positive Clinitest reaction. Crash dieting may be the cause of ketones in the urine.
5 Sugar and ketones in the urine may indicate uncontrolled diabetes mellitus.
6 To identify on laboratory examination whether urinary tract infection is present and to count the numbers of cells present. According to

Kass under 10,000 micro-organisms per ml of urine indicates absence of infection. Organisms grown from urine in the absence of pus cells indicates contaminated collection, 100,000 organisms per ml in three consecutive specimens indicates infection. The type of organism has to be identified. Pus cells are seen in nephritis and casts; red cells indicate haematuria which may be due to stones, infection, new growths. White cells present in large numbers indicate infection. If a midstream specimen is collected during menstruation, the specimen will be contaminated with blood. Catheter specimens are not done unless absolutely necessary, as infection can be introduced.

7 Oliguria means a reduced urinary output. Anuria means no urine passed and is usually linked to suppression when the kidneys are not functioning. Polydipsia means excessive thirst, polyuria means large volume of urine passed.

8 To obtain a qualitative estimate of protein, hormones, glucose and electrolytes and to measure the volume and specific gravity of urine passed in 24 hours.

9 20–40 mgs/100 ml of blood.

10 The kidneys are not functioning efficiently.

11 Indicates fairly advanced renal drainage.

12 Proteinuria, hypoproteinaemia with generalized oedema. It may be idiopathic or secondary to renal disease.

13 Blood in the urine.

14 Acute nephritis, injury to the kidney, stones, tumours, bleeding diseases, acute pyelitis or cystitis, tuberculosis, enlarged prostate gland, anticoagulent drugs.

15 Bile in the urine indicates obstruction to the normal outflow of bile. The urine is dark green or brown.

16 Liver function tests, cholecystography. Barium meal cholangiography.

17 To examine the structure and the function of the urinary tract. Non-functioning kidneys will not excrete the contrast medium, no shadow will be shown.

18 To examine visually the interior of the urinary bladder.

19 To pass ureteric catheters via a cystoscope so that X-rays of the ureters, renal pelvis and calyces may be taken. An injection of contrast medium is made through the ureteric catheters to facilitate the X-rays. Specimens of urine can be obtained from either kidney during the process.

20 To examine the renal vessels following the injection of hypaque.

21 To obtain a specimen of kidney tissue from microscopic examination when diagnosis of the underlying condition is difficult.

22 Shock due to allergic reaction. There may be signs of respiratory distress, sweating and urticaria.

23 a Bed rest, removal of catheters when specimens of urine have been collected. Severe pain or persisting blood in the urine must be reported. Encourage fluids and observe the vital signs.

b Encourage additional fluids, observe especially if the person is elderly.

c Rest in bed for 24 hours, observe urine for blood and vital signs for alteration. Backache and persistent haematuria should be reported.

24 Frequency of micturition, small amounts passed, blood in urine, pain on passing urine. With pyelitis, there is severe backache. The temperature, pulse and respiratory rates increase.

25 a Visual examination of the bronchi with an instrument called a bronchoscope, specimens of tissue or washings may be taken and foreign bodies may be removed.

b An examination of the bronchial tree by X-ray after introducing radio opaque substance into the airway.

26 To identify causitive organisms of infection, malignant cells; casts may be seen in the sputum of asthma patients.

27 Bed rest, plenty of fluids, moist inhalations, ensure general comfort, oral decongestants and antibiotics may be given. The patient's colour, respirations and complaints of pain should be noted together with response to treatment.

28 Observation of vital signs, especially respiratory rate, chest movements and colour. Any deteriorations should be reported.

29 The state of the heart, strength of conduction, initiation of impulses, abnormal heart action. Abnormalities can be identified and dealt with before the patient manifests physical abnormalities.

30 Gives indication of inflammatory activity. E.S.R. may be done to monitor the progress of the patient.

31 Vital signs should be taken and if the pulse becomes weak or irregular, the doctor should be informed. The site of catheterization should be inspected for irritation or thrombosis.

32 Streptococcus viridans most commonly.

33 Indicative of infarction, gives an indication of the time of occurrence. S.G.O.T. rises quickly after infarction and returns to normal in about a week. S.L.D.H. rises more slowly and returns to normal in about 10 days.

34 A reduction in the oxygen carrying capacity of blood as a result of fewer erythrocytes in circulation or a decrease in the concentration of haemoglobin.

35 5,000,000/cu mm of blood or $4 - 6 \times 10^{12}$/litre.

36 a Microcytic hypochromic cells with reduced iron and haemoglobin.

b Macrocytic hyperchromic cells with reduced B_{12} and folic acid.

37 Depression of bone marrow resulting in deficiency of leucocytes, thrombocytes and erythrocytes.

38 Blood tests, gastric function tests, bone marrow tests and Schilling test on urine and faeces.

39 Absence of hydrochloric acid.

40 Usually in relation to duodenal ulcer.

41 a Blood in the stools indicating high gastro intestinal bleeding. The stools have a very loose consistency with an offensive odour.

    b Bleeding from the gastro-intestinal tract characterized by vomiting altered blood.

42 Visual examination of an organ with a hollow lighted instrument called an endoscope.

43 The oesophagus is examined with an oesophagoscope, the stomach with a fibroscope or gastroscope, the colon with a sigmoidoscope, the rectum with a proctoscope.

44 Barium swallow for the oesophagus, barium meal for the stomach, barium meal and follow through for the small intestine, barium enema for the colon.

45 Hidden blood in faeces.

46 Babinski's sign is present normally up to two years of age. In later years the sign is indicative of upper motor neurone disease.

47 A positive sign of meningeal irritation.

48 Electroencephalogram to assess brain activity, neurological tests, lumbar puncture to examine the cerebrospinal fluid. Other tests include arteriogram, encephalogram, ventriculogram, myelogram.

49 Vomiting, headache, rise in temperature, photophobia, neck rigidity, positive Kernig's sign.

50 Leucocytes 10,000 per cu/mm or $4-11 \times 10^9$/litre of blood, divided into granulocytes. (Neutrophils, eosinophils and basophiles.) Agranulocytes, limphocytes and monocytes.

51 An increase in white blood cells above normal.

52 A decrease in white blood cells below the normal number.

53 250,000–500,000 per cu/mm of blood or $150-400 \times 10^9$/litre.

54 An excess of hydrochloric acid.

5 THE NURSING PROCESS

The nursing process has received a considerable amount of publicity in recent years; it is difficult at the moment to pick up a textbook or nursing magazine without seeing reference to it somewhere.

The objective of this section is to describe the four basic components of the **nursing process.**

What is the nursing process?

It is a system of individualised or personalised care based on the specific needs of the patient.

Traditionally, nurses have tended to base nursing care on the medical model, the nursing plan, and this has been concentrated more on medical requirements and less on nurse-centred aspects of patient care. Organisation of patient care has tended to be routine-dominated and largely task-orientated.

This meant that the total care required by any one patient was fragmented into tasks, the responsibility for which was divided amongst the nursing team usually according to their level of training. In fact the needs of the patient were categorised into an hierarchical arrangement which usually meant that basic nursing care became largely the responsibility of the more junior members of the team.

The nursing process offers a means by which patient care can be planned and delivered according to the specific needs of each patient.

In order to implement the nursing process, nursing must:

 i move from a task-orientated to a patient-orientated approach to care.

 ii realise and appreciate that it has both a **dependent** and an **independent** function which need to be considered in relation to other professions with which nurses work.

iii be prepared to make decisions about nursing care and be accountable for those decisions.

The four basic components of the nursing process are:

Assessment	Gathering information about the patient in order to identify problems that have implications for nursing.
Planning	Prescribing a specific plan of care that includes goals and the nursing action to achieve them.
Implementation	Carrying out the planned nursing care.
Evaluation	Testing the outcome of nursing actions against the previously stated goals.

The four phases overlap and the process is both continuous and cyclical.

Patient involvement in each of the phases of the process should be maximal.

The nursing process differs from previous approaches to nursing care largely because:

  i information gathering follows a positive and systematic approach.
 ii nursing care plans are personalised, care is planned according to the specific needs of the specific patient.
iii objectives of care (goals) are clearly stated, so everyone including the patient knows the purpose of the planned activity.
 iv care plans are written, so that information can be shared and communicated to all those involved in the care. There should therefore be more continuity of care.
  v patient independence is promoted since fullest consideration is given in the plan to the patient's self-care ability.
 vi the effectiveness of nursing care is positively evaluated.

The nursing assessment

The nursing assessment, which is the first stage of the nursing process, involves collecting information about the patient in order that any problems can be identified. It is a more positive approach to information collection than perhaps has been practised in the past and usually involves **interviewing the patient or taking a nursing history.**

This is more than the rather random and unstructured interview that has traditionally been incorporated into the admission procedure in the past, and which usually only amounted to some patients being asked some questions, sometimes. **The nursing history provides a systematic method of interviewing each patient so that all relevant information needed to effectively plan an individualised approach to care can be obtained.**

Many hospitals have devised their own questionnaire or checklist for this purpose and the information to be elicited usually includes details of the patient's social, cultural and economic background, past and present medical history (from the patient's point of view), physical and psychological condition.

This information may be collected from a variety of sources:

a the patient
b relatives or companions
c the patient's case notes
d the nursing observations
e the medical history and examination
f the nursing report or Kardex

The availability of such information depends upon exactly when the assessment is carried out and the ability of the patient to participate in the interview. Ideally, the nursing history should be taken as soon after the admission as possible, but to be realistic, much depends on the state of the ward, general nursing activity and staffing levels and the immediate care the patient might need.

In the planned admission situation, it might be possible to incorporate the nursing interview into the admission 'procedure'. In the emergency situation, when the patient requires immediate medical intervention, this might not be possible until later. In this instance, however, it is obvious that the patient is still continuously assessed, his immediate problems identified and nursing action given appropriate to and alongside the emergency medical intervention.

The time and method of taking the history, the type of documentation to be used and the question of who will take the history will therefore be determined at ward level.

When all the relevant information has been gathered, and after it has been checked for omissions and inconsistencies, a statement of the patient's problems is made.

Each statement should be clear and concise and where possible should include details about the cause or causes of the problem as well as the problem itself.

> e.g. **Restricted mobility** . . . problem
> due to osteo-arthritis of both hips,
> and old injury to right shoulder.
> Finds it particularly difficult to
> get up out of bed and to dress each
> morning.

This makes it quite clear to all that one patient's restricted mobility is quite different from any other patient's limitation.

The nurse, because of her theoretical knowledge and experience, makes inferences about the information she has gathered, considers a range of possibilities and predicts what will follow. As a result of this approach, she is able to identify problems and also put them into order of priority. The problems she might identify may be:

a **Actual**
b **Potential**
c **Possible**

A statement of the patient's problems is not a statement of the medical diagnosis, but rather of how the medical diagnosis (disease process) may be affecting the patient. Consequently, it is a statement of those factors concerning the patient which have implications for nursing actions.

e.g. The medical diagnosis may be:
Chronic bronchitis with acute exacerbation.

Medical diagnosis
Chronic bronchitis with acute exacerbation

Patient's problems
1 Breathlessness on the slightest exertion.
2 Dependency on others for daily living activities.
3 Left lower chest pain on coughing.
4 Difficulty in sleeping due to breathlessness.
5 Loss of appetite. Finds the taste of sputum puts him off his food.

These are **actual** problems, pertaining to the patient's present situation. As a result of the information available, and perhaps because of the actual problems identified, the nurse might be able to predict potential problems.
e.g. **Pressure sore formation** due to restricted mobility, thin and poorly nourished state.
Dehydration due to nausea and reluctance to drink.
The nurse might also infer that there may be **possible problems,** but would usually need more information from the patient or other sources before the existence of such problems can be verified.
Some problems may be solved within minutes of identifying them, some problems require no nursing intervention. Before planning care, the nurse should validate the existence of all problems and might need to return to the patient to do this.
Information has been gathered, problems have been identified, validated and clearly stated. The nurse is now in a position to plan her patient's care.

Planning
This involves the formulation of a **care plan** which is aimed at solving the patient's problems.
Once the patient's problems have been **identified and clearly stated** the nurse is in a position to **plan the specific care** which the patient requires in order to solve his or her problems.
The first step is to **define a goal for each of the problems identified.** The goal, like the problem, should be clearly and concisely stated and should contain two elements:
 i It should be patient centred; this means that the goal should relate to the desired response or activity of the patient.
 ii It should be capable of measurement or evaluation.
The following are examples of **goals:**
a The patient will be able to cope with the activities of bedrest with minimum breathlessness.
b The skin on pressure areas will remain intact and of normal colour.

c The patient will drink 2 litres in 24 hours.

All of the above goals relate to the patient, not the nurse's activity, and all lend themselves to evaluation.

Because the goals are stated in specific terms, the nurse can see whether they have been achieved or not.

They may be short-term or long-term goals but most important, they must be **realistic.**

Once the goals have been defined, the nurse should consider the most appropriate nursing actions that will lead to their achievement.

e.g.
Problem
Dehydration due to nausea and reluctance to drink.

Goal
Will drink 2 litres in 24 hours.

Nursing action
Explain the need for adequate fluid intake so as to obtain the patient's co-operation. Show him the goals and ask him to keep a written record of his fluid intake. Find out what drinks the patient likes and record them on the fluid chart. Provide drinks of the patient's choice and place within reach. Offer mouthwashes 2-hourly, after expectoration of sputum and before meals. Offer facilities for cleaning dentures 4-hourly. Check fluid intake at 12 mid-day and 4 p.m. Adjust intake accordingly.

At this stage in the planning, the nurse should decide when to review or evaluate each problem to see if the goals are being achieved.

The patient, whenever possible, should be fully involved in the planning stage since involvement in the planning of his own care promotes his fullest involvement and interest in the implementation of the plan.

Implementation
This is the actual giving of the planned nursing care and involves carrying out instructions from the medical staff and nursing instructions, within both the framework of prevailing hospital policies and the procedures that act as guidelines for hospital staff.

Organisation of nursing care has to be considered within the constraints of the typical ward situation. Some of the constraints are as follows:

a The workload generated by specific numbers of patients, their general conditions, their levels of dependency and the care they require at any given time.

b The structure or geography of the ward, available facilities for the provision of nursing care, e.g. equipment, ward stock levels.

c The availability and abilities of the care team, i.e. staff/patient ratios, and the levels of knowledge and expertise of individual members of the team.

Organisation of nursing care therefore involves:
i Assessment of the situation
e.g. Numbers of patients
    Levels of dependency of patients
    Nature of care required by patients
    e.g. pre-operative preparation, wound care,
        lifts and position changes
        Number of nurses on duty
        Levels of training or expertise of nurses

Ward activity:
e.g. doctor's rounds
    admissions
    discharges/transfers/departmental visits
    nurses needed for escort duties
    any other activities that have implications for nursing or require nursing involvement.

ii Organisation of the workload
'What needs to be done?'
'When should it be done?'
Too often nurses perform tasks simply because they have always been performed. They should question their nursing actions and they should be able to justify them.
e.g. 'All the beds must be made before 10 a.m.'
What is the reason for this? If there are no other priorities for nursing action, it might be reasonable for all the beds to be made by 10 a.m. However, one can argue that because of such rigid rules bedmaking might, and often does, take priority over patient care.
'All patients have their TPRs recorded at 6 a.m. and 6 p.m.'
What is the reason for this? If the reason is not a valid one, it means that valuable nursing time is taken up performing tasks that are not necessary. This could be seen as a waste of nursing resources.
The nurse needs to take an overview of the ward's total activity within the particular span of duty she is concerned with. She then needs to identify her priorities for nursing care in order to answer the questions of what needs to be done and when it should be done.
In the present type of system the nurse needs to consider such questions

within the constraints of the timed events which are difficult to change: i.e. meal times, shift change-overs.
This brings the nurse on to:

iii Delegation of duties
The nurse must consider who in the ward team is best able to deal with the particular nursing care responsibilities considered above.
When delegating responsibility the nurse in charge has to consider the **amount** and **level** of responsibility she should give to any individual.
She has to consider whether she wants each nurse to work alone, with a partner, in teams and also whether to task-allocate or patient-allocate the nursing care responsibility to her nurses.
Patient allocation is obviously the most desirable since there is less likelihood of each patient's care being fragmented, therefore allowing the nurse to consider the total care each patient requires. Patient allocation works without the 'Nursing Process', but the 'Nursing Process' cannot work without patient allocation.
Before the nursing care previously planned can be carried out the nurse in charge has to organise the ward so that **each nurse is aware of her specific responsibilities.**
The benefits of a written care plan can, at this implementation stage, be fully appreciated by the nursing care team.
Every member is aware of what needs to be done, why it needs to be done and what ends are to be achieved.

Evaluation
At the planning stage, the decision should have been made regarding when to evaluate specific aspects of care.
Evaluation can be seen as **assessing the patient's progress or otherwise in relation to achieving the goals that have been defined.**
In doing this the **quantity** and **quality** of care given may need to be questioned. This may be on a general basis or related to an individual nurse's performance.
For example:
> Have the goals been achieved?
> If not, were the goals realistic?
> If not, they need to be changed.
> If they are found to be realistic, were the nursing instructions effective towards achieving the goal?
> If not, they need to be changed.
> If they are considered to be effective, why were they not carried out?

Was the responsibility delegated appropriate to the level of knowledge and expertise of the individual member of staff?

This positive approach to evaluating nursing care can sometimes prove to be quite traumatic to the nursing staff, but nurses must be prepared to be self critical, they must be prepared to look inward, they must be willing to be accountable for the decisions about nursing care they have to make.

6 HELPING THE PATIENT WITH RESPIRATORY PROBLEMS

The objectives for the following chapters (6–12) are to:
1 Establish the individuality of the person in hospital.
2 Discuss how individuals may be helped with problems of respiration, excretion, eating, drinking, sleeping, pain and mobility.
3 To help students to test their knowledge and application in all the above areas.

Please use text books and lecture notes in conjunction with these chapters and refer to the respiration section in the chapter on vital signs and investigations.

Recognising the problem

The objectives of this section are concerned with identifying problems of respiration and helping the individual cope with these problems.

An individual is a unique centre of consciousness, usually in a balance of mind and body that is normal for him. When an individual arrives in hospital it is because something has happened to upset the balance. Pathological processes manifest themselves as signs or symptoms that may be physical or psychological (disease), altering the patient's life style to a greater or lesser degree. The level of dependency of an individual experiencing respiratory problems rests on the severity of the condition. The young fit man suffering from an upper respiratory tract infection will have different needs from the elderly person who suffers from emphysema or corpulence. The more severe the condition the greater the dependency will become. However fit the individual is at the onset of the disease, difficulty in breathing causes anxiety and a fear of the consequences that may not be overtly expressed. Every effort should be made to explain his symptoms clearly and to reassure him that his anxieties are recognised, otherwise the respiratory conditon may be exacerbated by frustration and anxiety creating an increased demand for oxygen.

The aims of nursing care are directed to long and short term goals.

1 To help the patient cope with his problems.
2 To help the patient breathe more easily by
   a Positioning the patient comfortably to facilitate rest and maximum ventilation.
   b Relief of pain.
   c Encouraging independence and mobility.
   d Preventing avoidable complications.
   e Maintaining or improving the level of dependency.

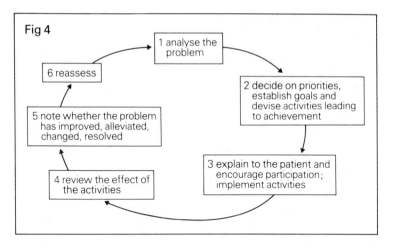

Fig 4

The first priority is to assess the degree of respiratory disability. The rate, rhythm and character of breathing is observed, together with the movements of the chest. The ease of breathing is observed e.g. does the individual stop for breath in the middle of sentences, does he purse his lips and blow out on expiration, does he have to use accessory muscles of respiration. Are abnormal breath sounds evident, or cyanosis, or flushing, does the person appear to be in pain. Is the temperature raised, or are there alterations in pulse rate and rhythm or blood pressure that may be significant? There are two kinds of information to be discussed:

i How the patient perceives his problem in relation to mobility, sleeping, eating, eliminating, socialising, and what the patient does to cope with his problem, e.g. how does he make his life easier, does he sleep downstairs in bed or in a chair, can he walk upstairs? Is he able to dress without difficulty, or does he need to rest during dressing? Does he need to sit after rising from bed to try to get his breath, can he walk to the toilet? How does he manage acute attacks, does he use drugs to relieve breathing, or an inhaler? Does he take oxygen at home?

ii How you perceive the patient's level of dependence so that realistic goals can be set to help the patient breathe more easily and cope with his situation.

The diagram above may be of help in setting goals and evaluating the outcome of the planned activities.

Steps to ensure comfortable and maximum ventilation

1 Individuals with fever and acute respiratory tract conditions are usually put into bed in a comfortable sitting position to ensure rest, warmth, and maximum ventilation. Occasionally patients with long term conditions of the respiratory tract state a preference to sit in a comfortable arm chair. If this is the case provision should be made to keep the individual warm and safe.

2 Aids to prevent pressure and provide support include bed-cradles sheepskins, foam pieces, ripple beds, back supports, and bed-table with pillow.

3 Exercises to improve circulation and respiration should be commenced, giving an explanation of why they are necessary and how they should be performed. Deep breathing and coughing of secretions into a sputum container are effective means of eliminating secretions. Removal of tenacious secretions can be assisted by gentle clapping of the chest with the cupped hand, occasionally postural drainage may be necessary to drain secretions from the lungs.

4 Moist inhalations or humidification and suction are useful in helping to remove tenacious mucous.

5 Oxygen therapy is given as prescribed by the doctor.

6 Expectorants and bronchodilators may be prescribed.

7 Assisted ventilation in the short term may be achieved by passing an endotracheal tube. For longer term duration and more efficient access to bronchial secretions tracheostomy is performed.

The patient should be actively encouraged to participate in his treatment, adapt to his condition and be independent. Assistance is given as necessary. Associated anorexia or constipation should be recognised, together with abnormal sleep patterns and steps should be taken to help improve these functions.

Practice Questions

1 What are the dangers of oxygen therapy?
2 What does hypoxia mean?
3 What do the terms hypercapnia and hypocapnia describe?
4 What does respiratory insufficiency mean?
5 Why are expectorants prescribed?
6 Why are cough suppressants prescribed?
7 What do diminished, sucking and paradoxical movements of the chest indicate?
8 What does the term cyanosis imply?
9 What information should be obtained on admission excluding name, address, age, religion, next of kin, and telephone number and name of doctor?
10 What investigations may be made to establish disease processes in the respiratory tract?
11 What are the dangers of bed rest?
12 Why are bronchodilators prescribed?
13 Why are broad spectrum antibiotics administered?
14 Describe the activities involved in suctioning.
15 Why is postural drainage carried out?
16 What factors are thought to predispose to chronic respiratory conditions?
17 What does tracheostomy mean?
18 For what reasons is tracheostomy performed?
19 What information can be obtained from inspecting sputum?
20 What do the terms respiratory emphysema and cor pulmonale mean?
21 What is the purpose of humidification?
22 What does the term pneumonia describe?
23 What does pleural effusion mean, give causes of pleural effusion.
24 Describe the care required by a person admitted to hospital with acute respiratory tract infection for the first 24 hours of hospitalisation.
25 What does atelectasis mean?
26 What does empyema mean?

Answers

1 The dangers of oxygen therapy are physical and physiological. Physical danger is fire. Oxygen supports combustion, therefore smoking or equipment which produces static electricity, or inflammable liquids should be prohibited in an area where oxygen is being used. Physiological dangers are drying and crusting of mucus membranes, particularly in relation to tracheostomy and carbon dioxide narcosis. Carbon dioxide provides 'drive' for the respiratory centre. For patients with chronic respiratory diseases, the respiratory centre becomes dependent on higher levels of CO_2 in the blood,

oxygen therapy may reduce the 'drive' by removing the stimulus. An irreversible condition of the eyes can occur in premature babies as a result of too high oxygen pressures, blindness ensues. Very occasionally individuals become claustrophobic and unable to tolerate oxygen masks.

2 Hypoxia means deficiency of oxygen in the tissues, and may result from arterial, anaemic, metabolic or circulatory causes.

3 Hypercapnia describes retention of carbon dioxide in the blood which may result from respiratory insufficiency, there may be changes in the activities of the lungs, kidneys, or circulatory system as a result. Hypocapnia describes decreased carbon dioxide in the blood, usually due to hyper-ventilation.
Respirations become slow and deep and, if of a long term, alkalosis and confusion results.

4 Respiratory insufficiency occurs when the individual is no longer able to maintain the levels of PCO_2 and PO_2 that are normally present.

5 To liquify secretions and make elimination easier.

6 To depress the cough reflex when the patient has an unproductive cough that is exhausting him.

7 Diminished movement of the chest wall on one side may be evident in pneumothorax or collapse of lung. Sucking movements of the chest may be seen when there is extreme difficulty in inspiration or expiration, paradoxical movements of the chest may be seen in chest injuries, i.e. 'flail chest' and therefore chest movement is an important observation in respiratory tract conditions.

8 Cyanosis is associated with excessive de-oxygenation of haemoglobin. Is usually associated with respiratory tract deficiencies and cardiac conditions.

9 Information to be obtained should relate to:
   a The patient's perception of his condition and the way he deals with it.
   b Housing accommodation, numbers of people occupying the accommodation, toilet facilities, bathing facilities, heating.
   c Attendance.
   d General nutritional state.
   e Whether the patient is able to maintain occupation.
   f What you perceive the patient's problem to be on admission.

10 Chest X-Ray, bacteriological and cytological examination of sputum. Respiratory function tests. Blood gases analysis. Full blood count. Bronchoscopy and biopsy or bronchography may be necessary. If pleural effusion is present it may be necessary to tap the fluid to relieve breathing and to obtain specimen of the fluid for examination in the laboratory. It may be necessary to take a specimen of pleura for histological examination.

11 Pressure, deep vein thrombosis, urinary stasis, hypostatic pneumonia, joint stiffness, loss of muscle tone.

12 Bronchodilators dilate the bronchial tubes by relaxing the smooth muscle, thus relieving breathing and helping elimination of secretions.

13 Broad spectrum antibiotics are given to protect the patient prior to determining the causative organism from the respiratory tract secretions.

14 Suctioning is done to remove secretions from the respiratory tract when the patient is unable to expectorate, or if secretions are tenacious. The nurse's hands must be washed and sterile gloves are put on. A sterile catheter is attached to the wall suction unit, the tip is exposed and is introduced gently into the respiratory tract. Precautions must be taken to avoid damaging the mucosa. Quite often introducing the catheter causes the patient to cough resulting in aspiration of deeper secretions. The catheter should be large enough to enable removal of thick secretions. If the catheter is to be passed through an endotracheal or tracheostomy tube it must be smaller than the lumen of the tube. Observe the type and volume of secretions aspirated. Use a sterile catheter for each suctioning.

15 Postural drainage is important in aiding the elimination of respiratory secretions that may cause collapse of lung or infection if they were retained. The patient is helped into a position so that secretions flow out by gravity. It may be necessary to administer bronchodilators beforehand and to assist by gently clapping the chest. The patient is encouraged to cough.

16 Cold damp climate, damp housing, overcrowding. Frequent attacks of respiratory infections. Irritants in the atmosphere, i.e. air pollutants and cigarette smoking. Heredity may play a part.

17 An artificial opening in the trachea.

18 Tracheostomy is done to relieve airway obstruction, to remove tracheo bronchial secretions and to give assisted respiration when the patient cannot maintain respiratory efficiency, as in respiratory insufficiency, head injuries, poliomyelitis, etc.

19 Watery sputum may be seen in pneumonia, purulent sputum in bronchiectasis, tenacious sputum in chronic respiratory disease, blood stained or rusty sputum is seen in pneumonia, green or yellow sputum indicates infection, haemoptysis may result from pulmonary tuberculosis or carcinoma of lung. Volume raised is important.

20 Respiratory emphysema usually results from chronic respiratory disease. The alveoli dilate and several air sacs join to form one large space. Loss of alveoli results in poor ventilation and exchange of gases is impeded, thus there is an increase in PCO_2 and decrease in PO_2. Cor pulmonale is respiratory disease secondary to heart disease.

21   Humidification increases the moisture in inspired air. An aerosol mist is helpful in helping to eliminate thick secretions from the respiratory tract.

22   Pneumonia implies inflammation of lung tissue. Lobar pneumonia refers to an affected lobe, segmental pneumonia refers to an affected segment, bronchial pneumonia refers to disease occuring in patches in one or both lungs.

23   A collection of fluid between the parietal and visceral pleura. A large accumulation will embarrass breathing. An effusion may be due to increased venous pressure in heart and liver disease, or infection or malignant disease.

24   The patient should be placed in bed in a comfortable sitting position, well supported. Physical and mental rest are important to his well-being. Explanations of treatment should be clearly made with every attempt to reduce anxiety. Pressure areas should be protected and movement encouraged, together with breathing exercises. Observation of vital signs should be recorded as frequently as necessary, together with movements of the chest. If significant alterations in chest movements are observed, this should be reported. A low blood pressure and falling temperature, together with a raised pulse and respiratory rate should be reported, as shock or spread of infection may be indicated. Changes in colour, pallor or cyanosis should be reported and signs of disorientation. Sputum should be inspected for characteristics and volume.
Fluids should be given freely, and fluid balance should be recorded. Nutrition is given in the form of liquid foods. Mouth care is important as is attention to general hygiene. A laxative or suppository may be necessary to relieve constipation.
Medical management
A full blood count will be taken, with blood gas analysis, and chest X-ray. Humidified oxygen is usually prescribed. While the cough is unproductive, a cough suppressant is usually ordered to prevent exhaustion. Chest pain may be relieved by warmth and an analgesic. A broad spectrum antibiotic is usually ordered.

25   Atelectasis means collapse of part of or a lobe of the lung usually following obstruction of a bronchial tube by a plug of mucus.

26   Empyema is a collection of pus in an organ.

7 HELPING THE PATIENT WITH EXCRETION OF WASTES AND BODY FLUID

When an individual arrives at hospital, enquiries should be made about patterns of micturition and defaecation. The individual's age, culture or preconceived ideas about hospitalisation could cause problems regarding elimination, and anxieties may be resolved if discussed at the initial interview.

It should be remembered that when an individual meets a potentially stressful situation, nervous reaction could cause sweating, vomiting, frequency of micturition or diarrhoea. These effects are usually of a transient nature and may be resolved by recognition of nervousness so that reassurance may be given.

The aims of nursing care with regard to the objective should be
1 To relieve stress and anxiety
2 To help relieve discomfort
3 To help relieve pain
4 To prevent avoidable complications
5 To maintain or improve the level of dependence
6 To observe the frequency of elimination and type of material eliminated
7 To note significant changes that may be of vital importance to the well-being of the patient.

Micturition and defaecation

Individuals coming into hospital will be apprehensive. The thought of a rigid hospital routine, sharing communal facilities, could provoke anxiety. Some people may have ritualistic attitudes to elimination, others may consider enquiries about elimination habits to be an invasion of privacy. Normal patterns should be elicited at interview and as far as possible, anxieties should be relieved.

On admission all patients able to walk should be shown the toilet facilities. It may be necessary to reassure individuals about the cleanliness of communal facilities. Some may fear infection. If paper seat covers are not available advise the use of paper towels as seat covers. For some individuals it may be necessary to demonstrate the flush, or explain to others how the toilet is used.

For individuals who are unable to walk, a sanichair may be provided as transport to the lavatory, this is more satisfactory than having to use a commode or bedpan. However, it may be that a commode or bedpan is the alternative. Individuals who until the onset of illness have managed the process of excretion with privacy and without help, will feel embarrassed or possibly inhibited at having to relieve themselves in the ward. Keep the above points in mind and:

a Ensure privacy at all times whether helping the patient in the lavatory or in the ward.

b Help the disabled individual to adopt the position for excretion which is most comfortable and effective for them.

c If necessary make sure the skin is clean and dry after excretion.

d Provide hand washing facilities, it may be necessary to train some individuals in hygiene.

e If a commode or bedpan has been used remove immediately after helping the patient to attend to hygiene.

f Use an air freshener to deodorise the area if necessary.

g Report abnormalities in urine or faeces.

Micturition

Some points for nursing observation with regard to micturition. Frequency of micturition may result from nervousness, cold, increased fluid intake or treatment with diuretics not usually associated with pain.

Refer to chapter on investigations for
abnormal volume and constituents of urine

Infection in the urinary tract is usually associated with pain: irritation of the bladder mucosa results in frequency, urgency and pain. Frequency may be associated with stones in the bladder, or pressure from a pregnant uterus.

Retention

Retention of urine is commonly caused by bladder neck or urethral obstruction, it may occur after surgery in the immediate post-operative period, it is associated with spinal injuries, diseases of the nervous system and may occur in labour. The individual experiencing urine retention has the desire to urinate and tries without effect to empty the bladder. The bladder distends, becomes obviously palpable, there is increasing discomfort and pain with restlessness, sweating and tachycardia. Retention with overflow often occurs in long standing retention when the sphincter is forced open and urine dribbles out. Changing the individual's position may help the patient to pass urine, e.g. sitting up on a bedpan or commode, running water over the pubic area, whistling, running tap water, helping a man stand upright, sharp drinks or a warm bath may all be effective in helping relieve the patient. If all attempts to help the patient urinate fail carbachol may be ordered or catheterisation. If the retention is of long standing only 1000 ml of urine is released after catheterisation, to be followed by slow decompression of the bladder. Whether the catheter is to remain in the bladder or to be open or closed drainage depends on the condition of the individual. Where there is spinal injury an automatic bladder may be established so that urinary retention may be relieved by pressure over the pubic area.

Incontinence

Incontinence means involuntary passing of urine. This may occur as a result of the degeneration process, it may be associated with neurological disease or injury. It can occur after prostatectomy or long standing catheterisation, the latter usually responds to exercises in bladder control. The skin, if constantly wet and irritated by urine, will break; in an effort to prevent this the incontinent person must be kept clean and dry, appliances can be used to collect urine, or the person may be catheterised. Catheterisation is a potential hazard. The genital area must be clean and the catheter should be cleaned to prevent ascending infection.

Stress incontinence usually occurs in lax pelvic floor muscles, when the individual laughs or coughs urine is passed involuntarily. This is potentially embarrassing and until the condition is rectified with a pessary or repair, absorbent pads may relieve the individual of psychological stress temporarily.

Suppression of urine means no urine is formed, as in acute renal failure, or only a few mls of urine are passed in 24 hours.

Deviations of urinary drainage

Congenital abnormalities or removal of urinary bladder necessitates transplantation of ureters either into the colon or the ileum. For the former procedure no external appliance is necessary as the anal sphincter controls the output of very soft faeces and urine. For the latter procedure the care is similar to that of the ileostomy patient with regard to care of stoma, skin, changing appliances, fluid balance, replacement of fluids and psychological support of the person.

Defaecation

The normal pattern of bowel habit should be elicited at initial interview. Some individuals may have diarrhoea due to nervousness. This should abate when they settle in. Some individuals are extremely bowel conscious and become very concerned if they do not evacuate the bowel at least once in 24 hours. Other individuals habitually take aperients on which they become dependent for a bowel action. Factors that cause constipation in hospital may be the following.

a Pain on defaecation.
b Inhibition at having to use communal facilities.
c Alteration in diet or reduced fluid intake.
d Lack of exercise or being in the recumbent position.
e Withdrawal of aperients taken habitually so that tone and peristalsis of the intestine is ineffective.

f Some drugs may cause constipation by reducing peristalsis.

g Constipation is usually associated with fever.

Constipation may be a feature of abnormalities of the intestine or disease in the intestine; it may also be associated with general disease e.g. myxoedema.

Constipation

The cause of the constipation should be identified.

Nursing management and aims are

i To relieve distress and discomfort. Constipation if habitual can damage the rectal mucosa, straining at stool may cause haemorrhoids.

ii To explain why the urge to defaecate should be obeyed.

iii To explain how a high fibre diet can help.

iv To explain the importance of exercise, if exercise is possible.

v To explain why aperients should not be taken habitually.

It may be necessary initially to relieve constipation by giving a strong aperient or suppository until evacuation is achieved. Faecal impaction may be relieved by giving olive oil enema followed by an evacuent enema. Manual removal of faeces may be necessary; this should be done with care as it is a procedure that may cause the patient to faint.

Diarrhoea

Diarrhoea may be a sign of nervousness, may be a symptom of disease in the intestine or general disease such as thyrotoxicosis. Changes in diet, e.g. spicy food, may cause diarrhoea, or infected food. Drugs may irritate the mucosa or destroy the normal flow of the intestine leaving it unprotected. Antibiotics are an important group of drugs having an effect on the intestine.

The cause of diarrhoea should be identified if possible.

Nursing management of an individual with diarrhoea.

a If infection is suspected, the patient should be barrier nursed and the stools should be disinfected before disposal.

b The patient with acute diarrhoea should be kept at rest as frequent stools and loss of body fluid is exhausting. Depending on the general state of the patient, oral or intravenous fluids may be given. If the patient is debilitated he should be assisted on and off the bedpan or commode. Make sure the patient's skin is kept clean and dry. If the person has acute diarrhoea the anal area becomes sore, creams may be applied. If a fissure in ano is present local anaesthetic ointment may relieve the pain after defaecation.

c Observe the patient's condition, the type of stool, volume and number passed in 24 hours.

d Drugs are ordered to treat infection, or to slow down the activity of the bowel. The patient's response to treatment should be noted.

Coughing

A cough is an involuntary response to an irritant in the respiratory tract, or to pressure from outside the respiratory tract, less commonly it may be psychogenic or an attention seeking device. The cause of the cough should be identified, if possible.

The nursing management and aims.

a Rest the patient with an unproductive cough, usually cough suppressants are ordered to prevent exhaustion.

b Encourage the patient with a productive cough to raise sputum.

c Observe whether the patient needs help with expectoration.

   i Support head or painful part, encourage deep breathing exercises.

   ii Hold sputum carton.

   iii Humidification and moist inhalation can help relieve tenacious secretions. Aerosol administration of mucolytic enzymes help liquefy secretions.

   iv Gentle clapping of the chest may release tenacious sputum, postural drainage may be necessary to help secretions flow out by gravity.

   v Observe reaction to expectorants ordered, or to bronchodilators.

   vi Observe volume and character of sputum raised.

   vii Encourage prevention of infection by following physiotherapist's instructions and by disposal of paper handkerchiefs correctly and closing sputum carton after use.

Refer to chapter on vital signs and investigations.

Sweating

Sweating makes a person feel uncomfortable and self-conscious. Depending on the cause of sweating, a person may take a bath, or may have to be blanket bathed. The aim should be to make the person comfortable and to prevent chilling. The cause of sweating should be identified.

Sweating may be due to anxiety or nervousness which is relieved when the individual is reassured. Sweating is a common feature of the menopause, thyrotoxicosis and shock; it may be associated with pain or with raised body temperature, or with increased activity, or changes in environmental temperature. It may be necessary to tepid sponge or cool the patient. It is important to remember:

a Not to chill sweating patients.

b After sponging or drying change damp clothing.

c To adjust the temperature to a comfortable level.

d To provide an electric fan if needed.

e To give fluids if allowed.

f To observe whether sweating is diminishing.

g To place damp clothes in a clothing bag to avoid soiling clean clothing.

h To record temperature after sponging.
Refer to the chapter on vital signs for control of body temperature.

Vomiting
Vomiting may be caused by nervousness, or it may be a feature of infection, or disease, or obstruction in the gastro-intestinal tract. The origin of vomiting may be emotional or psychogenic, or result from incompatible food or drugs, or neurological disease.
The cause of vomiting should be identified.

Nursing management of the vomiting patient

a The most comfortable and safe position should be adopted. If the patient is conscious and able to sit up a denture carton, vomit bowl and paper handkerchiefs should be provided. Support the patient's head and painful parts and remove dentures. If the patient is unable to sit up, the lateral position is best so that the patient's head can be supported over the vomit bowl. When vomiting has ceased a mouthwash should be offered, change linen if necessary and leave a covered vomit bowl at hand. If the patient is unconscious, the semi-prone position is safest; ensure the airway is not obstructed, remove dentures, and use suction to clear away debris. Clean the mouth when vomiting has ceased. The danger of vomiting in the unconscious person is asphyxiation or aspiration of vomit into the lungs, especially if the position is not effective, or suction is ineffective.

b Encourage the nauseated patient to take deep breaths; this may prevent vomiting. Ensure rest and quiet.

c Note the volume, characteristics and frequency of vomiting, or the stimulus with which it is associated.

d If you think anxiety is the cause of vomiting, try to get the patient to voice his worry.

e It may be necessary to pass a nasogastric tube to relieve the patient of the chore of vomiting. The stomach should be aspirated at regular intervals. If vomiting occurs with a naso-gastric tube in position, this may mean i. The tube is out of position, ii. The tube is obstructed. i. and ii. should be dealt with immediately. Observe whether the volume of aspirate is increasing or decreasing.

f When vomiting stops, the patient may be able to tolerate oral fluids. If vomiting is persistent, intravenous fluids will be given.

g Accurate measurement of fluid balance must be maintained.

h If anti-emetic drugs are prescribed the effect the drug has on the patient should be observed.

Wound drainage

The aim of wound drainage is to allow the escape of haemo-serous fluids, bile, pus or air so that wound healing proceeds with as little hindrance as possible. Uninfected wounds should heal by first intention.

Nursing management aims to facilitate wound drainage by

a Positioning the patient carefully so that drainage tubes are not pulled or obstructed or accidentally removed. If tubes are removed accidently before advised the medical officer should be informed immediately. It may be necessary to re-introduce the tube.

b Explaining to the patient why drainage tubes should not be touched. Helping the patient cope with wound drainage.

c Collecting the drained fluid into the appropriate bag or container, e.g. drainage bags, redivac bottles, underwater seal drainage.

d Observing the type and volume of fluid drained, noting significant abnormalities.

e Keeping accurate records.

f Protecting the skin so that it does not become sore or excoriated.

g Dealing with specific appliances such as redivac drainage and underwater seal drainage, and pumps which may be used to facilitate drainage.

h Keeping the wound dry.

i Milking drainage tubes to encourage free draining.

j Shortening tubes daily so that wounds heal from below up to the surface.

k Observing the individual's condition generally while attending to drainage.

l Taking precautions as in chest drainage to clamp the chest tube while helping the patient to move, making sure that clamps are removed when the individual is repositioned. Keeping an airtight dressing available so that the puncture wound can be sealed if the tubes are accidentally removed.

m Following the advice of doctors and the rules of the procedure committee regarding the well-being of a patient with wound drainage.

Practice Questions

 1 What does dysuria mean?
 2 What does micturition mean?
 3 State the symptoms of urine retention.
 4 Describe the symptoms of bladder infection.
 5 State the treatment of bladder infection.
 6 What does incontinence mean?
 7 Why does urinary overflow occur with retention?
 8 What are the dangers of catheterisation?
 9 What are the dangers of incontinence of urine?
10 State the effects of habitually taking aperients.
11 What advice should be given to individuals with constipation?
12 State examples of drugs that reduce peristaltic action.
13 What may
    a loose green offensive stools
    b red current jelly stools
    c grey offensive stools or fatty stools
    in the infant or young child indicate?
14 What does melaena indicate?
15 What is the difference between a melaena stool and iron stool?
16 Give the meaning of defaecation.
17 What may bright red blood in the stool indicate?
18 What does the individual with carcinoma in the rectum complain of
    initially?
19 What may alternating bouts of diarrhoea and constipation indicate?
20 Name the common causative organisms of intestinal infection.
21 What would be an appropriate diet for a patient with diarrhoea?
22 What does diverticulitis mean, what symptoms are associated with it?
23 State the symptoms of Crohn's disease.
24 What treatment is given for control of Crohn's disease?
25 Describe the care needed by a patient with a productive cough.
26 How could you ensure that a patient with an unproductive cough
    rests?
27 What may the following indicate
    a Muco purulent sputum
    b Rusty sputum
    c Haemoptysis
    d Watery sputum
    e Offensive pus
28 What is the action of mucolytic enzymes?
29 Why is postural drainage necessary?
30 What does febrile mean?
31 What are the dangers of vomiting for the unconscious person?
32 What causes

    a Faeculent vomiting?
    b Projectile vomiting?
    c Haematemesis?
33 What is the function of a redivac drain?
34 What is the function of an underwater seal drain?
35 Why is it necessary to shorten a tube or corrugated drain daily?
    Answers
  1 Pain experienced on micturition.
  2 Passing urine.
  3 No urine passed though fluids are being taken. The urinary bladder distends. The desire to pass urine is constantly present, but attempts to pass urine are ineffective. The patient experiences increasing discomfort and pain; there is usually sweating, restlessness and tachycardia.
  4 Frequency, urgency and dysuria. There may be fever and blood and pus in the urine. Because the bladder mucosa is irritated small amounts of urine are passed.
  5 Bacterial examination of urine to identify causative organisms. Appropriate antibiotics or urinary antiseptics are ordered. Fluids are given and the patient is kept warm and rested.
  6 Loss of voluntary control of passing urine or faeces.
  7 Increased pressure in the urinary bladder forces the sphincter to partially open so that urine dribbles out.
  8 Ascending infection in the urinary tract. Traumatisation of meatal mucosa. Creation of a false passage in the male. Stretching of the sphincter in long standing catheterisation and loss of bladder tone.
  9 Excoriation of the skin, water-logging of skin causing breakdown and potential pressure sores.
10 Reduced peristalsis, loss of intestinal tone so that bowel evacuation is dependent on taking aperients in stronger doses.
11 Always obey the urge to defaecate. Try to establish a routine for bowel evacuation. Take a high fibre diet, take plenty of fluids and exercise. Avoid using aperients.
12 Opiates, e.g. Codeine. Anti-cholinergic drugs.
13 a Gasto-enteritis.
    b Intussusception.
    c Cystic fibrosis.
14 Bleeding high in the gastro-intestinal tract associated with peptic ulceration.
15 The melaena stool is loose, offensive and tarry, the stool from iron therapy is black and formed.
16 Evacuation of bowel.
17 It may be a sign of haemorrhoids bleeding at stool, or carcinoma in the rectum.

18 Usually of a feeling of fullness after defaecation.

19 Carcinoma in the colon.

20 Staphylacoccus, Salmonella, Shigella.

21 Fluids initially, followed by a low residue diet, with vitamin supplements.

22 Inflammation of a sac like structure on the intestinal wall, causing abdominal pain and diarrhoea.

23 Colicky abdominal pain, offensive diarrhoea, vomiting, weight loss, anaemia, anal fissures, skin lesions.

24 Salazopyrin, Lomotil, iron, codeine phosphate, systemic and local steroids.

25 Help the patient into a rested sitting position. Encourage chest physiotherapy and coughing at regular intervals.
Instruct the person in the use of sputum cartons. It may be necessary to give humidification or moist inhalations or mucolytic enzymes to release tenacious secretions. It may be necessary to assist removal of secretions by back clapping or postural drainage. Expectorants or bronchodilators may be ordered. General measures to ensure comfort must be given and general observations made of the patient's response to treatment.

26 Sit the patient in a comfortable position, avoid irritants like cigarette smoke, usually a cough suppressant, i.e. linctus, is ordered. An unproductive cough can exhaust the patient. The reaction of the patient to the treatment should be noted. Encourage relaxation and rest.

27 a Chest infection
  b Pneumonia
  c Infection i.e. tubercular, carcinoma of lung
  d Pulmonary oedema
  e Bronchiectasis

28 Liquefying of secretions in the respiratory tract to release tenacious sputum.

29 To help fluid out of the respiratory tract by placing the patient in positions so that secretions flow out by gravity. Usually postural drainage is proceeded by humidification expectorants and bronchodilators. Usually the nurse stays with the patient during these exercises.

30 Fever.

31 Asphyxiation, inhalation of vomit into the lungs.

32 a Advanced intestinal obstruction,
   b Hypertrophic pyloric stenosis,
   c Peptic erosion of an ulcer, gastric carcinoma, irritation of gastric mucosa with drugs or diet. Haematemesis may be due to swallowing of blood occasionally.

33 To remove secretions from a wound by vacuum.

34 To remove fluid and air from the pleural space after surgery or injury so that the lung may re-expand.

35 To allow the wound to heal from below, upwards.

8 HELPING THE PATIENT TO EAT AND DRINK

The need to eat and drink is a very basic one. Fulfilling the need is such an integral part of our lives that its importance is often taken for granted. It is only when we are unable to adequately meet the need that we begin to realise how fundamental eating and drinking is to our very existence. On the surface we tend to think of eating and drinking as the activity of feeding ourselves, ie. the action of putting food and fluids into our mouths, of swallowing, digesting and absorbing them. But, eating and drinking are far more complex activities than that; they have combined physical, psychological, social, cultural and even economic elements.

The motor skills involved in obtaining food, in going out and buying it, or growing it, in preparing it and eating it are many and varied; the mental skills involved in knowing what food is necessary, from where to obtain it, and how best to prepare it are influenced amongst other things by previous experience, general and educational background, by advice received personally or via the media, by levels of intelligence, powers of concentration and the desire to want to eat.

Eating and drinking are largely social events; they are mostly carried out in the company of others, meals at home are often timed so that the family can sit down together and are often the only times of the day when this might happen. At school, at work, and during leisure times, we tend to eat in groups; it is not difficult to understand the plight of the elderly person living alone who is able in other respects to prepare a meal but simply lacks the will to do so.

Cultural and religious backgrounds may impose certain restrictions on a diet, the effects of which will vary according to the mainstream culture and environment in which the smaller cultural group find themselves. For example, the anaemias and vitamin deficiency diseases are unfortunately increasing amongst the Asian immigrant population in the U.K. because of the inability, so far, to effectively 'marry' their dietary restrictions with the way of life and what food is available in this country (or vice versa).

Unfortunately food costs money, the cost is ever rising, the effects of inflation, together with the rise in unemployment, will no doubt further influence our choice of diet, our eating habits, and our nutritional status. We develop eating habits which best fit our particular life style or pattern. They might not be the most sensible habits, they might even be detrimental to our health in the long-term, nevertheless we are often reluctant to change them.

When a person is admitted to hospital, he becomes almost entirely dependent on the nursing staff, and to a lesser extent his visitors, for the selection, presentation and provision of his food and drink. Simply being in hospital regardless of the reason why, takes away his independence, being confined to bed limits him still further and in addition, because of the nature of his condition, he might be dependent on others to actually feed him.

There are very few hospitals that can provide the patient with the personal meal service he might have in his own home, but there are many hospitals that could provide a service more appropriate to the individual needs of each patient. The nursing staff spend more time with the patient than anyone else involved in his care. They work closely with the medical staff and other hospital personnel not only delivering care, but co-ordinating the care given by others. Meeting the patient's nutritional needs is an important part of this care and the nurse needs to consider her part in meeting this need alongside the part played by the catering department, the ward housekeeping/domestic team and possibly the dietician.

The responsibilities of the nursing staff with regard to helping the patient to eat and drink adequately are many and include the following:

1   In making a general assessment of the patient's needs, appropriate emphasis should be given to assessment of his nutritional status. This would obviously be considered in relation to the patient's general condition and the nature of the disease process/reason for hospitalisation. It would include finding out details of the patient's normal eating habits, his likes and dislikes, imposed dietary restrictions, his nutritional state at that point in time, e.g. underweight, obese, dehydrated, and how his particular condition/disease process interferes with his ability to eat and drink adequately and with his digestive/absorption capability.

2   In planning mealtimes, in helping the patient to cope with mealtimes (as well as in-between mealtimes), every consideration should be given to the patient's self-care ability. Provision of the most pleasant environment possible, of mealtimes disassociated from unpleasant procedures, adequate preparation of the patient; assisting him into the most comfortable position; the use of the most suitable eating utensils; affording him adequate time in which to eat his meal and providing him with appropriate assistance throughout, are some of the most important considerations.

3   Providing relevant information about dietary needs and dietary sources, giving adequate instruction to patients and their relatives about food content, preparation and hygiene; affording each patient the opportunity to discuss his dietary needs and perhaps even persuading him to take food and drink when he does not want to do so, are interpersonal skills which each nurse should develop.

4 Food should be attractively presented, it should be served at the correct temperature, with the most appropriate eating utensils available. The presentation should take into consideration the patient's choice of foods, his particular likes and dislikes with regard to the way it is served on his plate, and the size of the portion.

5 Mealtimes should be supervised so that the patient can be given assistance and encouragement when necessary, can be offered suitable alternatives should he fail for any reason to complete his meal. A record can them be made of the patient's dietary and fluid intake, and of his response, desirable or otherwise, to the food and drink taken.

6 When alternative methods of feeding the patient, e.g. nasogastric, gastrostomy, intravenous, are necessary, the nurse should be able to prepare the patient and equipment.
The nurse will either set up or assist the doctor to set up, the alternative route and care for the patient before, during and after the feed and/or administer the feed as appropriate.

7 Nursing staff should be able to discuss the nutritional needs of the patient with the patient, his relatives, the dietician, the catering and nursing staff, and the medical staff.

Practice Questions

1 Answer the following questions

a Describe briefly the act of swallowing.

b What are the functions of saliva?

c What are the four phases or activities performed by the digestive system?

d List (in order) the parts of the alimentary tract.

e What are the necessary organs of digestion?

f Describe briefly the functions of the stomach.

g What is the action of enterogastrone?

h What are the juices found in the small intestine?

i Distinguish between exocrine and endocrine functions of the pancreas.

j Differentiate between the absorption of fats, proteins and carbohydrates in the intestines.

k Name the nine descriptive regions of the abdomen.

l What observations/information should be noted when a patient has vomited.

m What are the signs and symptoms of dehydration?

n What are the functions of the following foodstuffs in our body:
   i   protein
   ii carbohydrates
   iii fats
   iv mineral salts
   v   vitamins

o What might be the complications of a neglected 'dirty' mouth?

p What extra-oral routes may be used to feed a patient?

2 What do you understand by the following terms

a Essential amino acid

b First class protein

c Metabolism

d Peyer's patches

e Peristaltic action

f Emaciation

g Cachexia

h Malnutrition

i Anorexia

j Enzyme

k Oesophageal reflux

l 'Drip and suck'

m Paralytic ileus

n Crypts of Leiberkuhn

o Achalasia
p Fractional test meal

3 Match the items a–l to the explanations in i–xii.
a Secretin
b Pepsinogen
c Enterokinase
d Maltase
e Pancreozymin
f Trypsinogen
g Cholecystokinin
h Salivary amylase
i Gastrin
j Lipase
k Pepsin
l Enterogastrone

   i an hormonal agent released by the small intestine and which stimulates pancreatic secretion.

   ii an hormonal agent released by the duodenum in response to the fat contents of chyme and which stimulates contractions of the gall bladder.

   iii commences the breakdown of cooked starch in the mouth.

   iv an hormonal agent released by the small intestine in response to the presence of food and which stimulates pancreatic secretion.

   v an hormonal agent which stimulates the secretion of gastric juices.

   vi an enzyme which converts proteins into smaller molecules in the stomach.

   vii released by the stomach as granules and is changed into a protein-splitting enzyme in the presence of hydrochloric acid.

   viii an enzyme found in pancreatic juice and which converts fats into fatty acids and glycerol.

   ix in response to fat in the food, this inhibits the activity of the stomach and thus delays emptying.

   x released by the small intestine and which activates trypsinogen in the pancreatic juice to form trypsin which contributes to the breakdown of proteins.

   xi an enzyme found in the cells lining the small intestine which continues the breakdown of disaccharides into monosaccharides.

   xii present in the pancreatic juice and needs to be activated to form trypsin in order to continue protein breakdown.

Answers

1 **a** Food taken into the mouth is masticated, mixed with saliva and formed into a bolus. The bolus is pushed backwards into the pharynx by the tongue which presses against the hard palate. The muscles of the pharynx contract and propel the bolus down into the oesophagus. (The bolus is prevented from **i** entering the nose by the elevation of the soft palate, **ii** returning to the mouth by the position of the tongue against the pillars of the fauces and **iii** the larynx by its elevation which brings its opening under the epiglottis.) The bolus then passes down the oesophagus into the stomach by peristaltic action. Breathing is inhibited until the latter stage of swallowing.

  b   i Lubrication of food in preparation for swallowing.
      ii Lubrication of mouth and teeth, thus helping speech.
      iii Facilitates sensation of taste — the taste buds on the tongue are stimulated by particles present in food which are dissolved in water.
      iv Cleansing action thus inhibiting the growth of bacteria.
      v Digestive — the enzyme ptyalin or salivary amylase acts upon starch.
      vi Excretion, many organic and inorganic substances are excreted in the saliva.

  c Ingestion, digestion, absorption, elimination.

  d Mouth, pharynx, oesophagus, stomach, duodenum, jejunum, ileum, ascending transverse and descending colon, sigmoid colon, rectum, anal canal.

  e Three pairs of salivary glands, parotid, submaxillary, submandibular.
    Pancreas.
    Liver and biliary tract.

  f   i Acts as a reservoir allowing time for mechanical and some chemical digestion to take place.
      ii Secretion of mucus which lubricates the passage of food.
      iii Secretion of gastric juice which begins the chemical digestion of proteins.
      iv Secretion of the hormone gastrin which stimulates the secretion of gastric juices.
      v Limited absorption of water, alcohol, glucose and some drugs.

When the contents of the stomach have reached the required consistency and degree of acidity, it is referred to as chyme. This is passed through into the duodenum in small amounts when the pyloric sphincter relaxes and the muscular stomach walls contract.

g This is a substance formed in the intestinal mucosa which is released in response to the fat content of food eaten and which exerts an inhibitary effect on both gastric secretion and motility — thus delaying emptying of the stomach.

h i Intestinal juice (succus entericus) which is alkaline in reaction, is secreted by the crypts of Lieberkuhn and contains digestive enzymes.

ii Pancreatic juice which also contains digestive enzymes.

iii Bile released from the gall bladder.

i The pancreas consists of a number of lobules, each of which is drained by a duct. These ducts unite with each other, eventually reach the main pancreatic duct which passes the whole length of the pancreas and joins with the termination of the common bile duct to enter the duodenum at the ampulla of Vater. The duodenal opening is controlled by the Sphincter of Oddi. **The exocrine secretion, pancreatic juice** which contains digestive enzymes, leaves the gland via the pancreatic duct. The presence of food in the small intestine releases the hormonal agents **secretin** and **pancreozymin** which stimulates this pancreatic secretion. Also found in the substance of the pancreas are collections of cells known as the **islets of Langerhans.** There are two types of cells, alpha cells which produce the hormone **glucagon,** whilst the beta cells produce **insulin. The secretion from the islets of Langerhans** is passed directly into the circulating blood and is **therefore the endocrine secretion.** Insulin facilitates the entry of glucose into the cells, **glucagon** raises the blood glucose level by mobilising **liver glycogen.**

j The surface area of the mucous membrane lining of the small intestine is greatly increased by the circular folds of mucous membrane and the finger-like projections called **villi.** The villi consist of a central lacteal surrounded by blood capillaries, the walls of the villi consist of epithelial cells through which absorption of substances from the intestinal lumen can take place.

Glucose and amino acids are absorbed into the blood capillaries of the villi and fatty acids and glycerol are absorbed into the central lacteal.

k Left hypochondrium   Epigastrium   Right hypochondrium
Left lumbar   Umbilical   Right lumbar
Left iliac   Hypogastric   Right iliac

l amount
consistency
colour   of vomit
smell

Was the patient nauseated before vomiting?

What was the nature of the vomiting? — projectile, retching, or was the vomitus regurgitated without effort.

How often is the vomiting occurring?

What time did the vomiting occur, can it be associated with anything else, e.g. food, drugs, position?

Are there any other symptoms, e.g. pain, headache?

What are the general effects on the patient?

m The signs and symptoms would obviously depend on the severity of the fluid deficit and the rate at which it developed but generally:

   i an early symptom would be thirst

   ii reduction of salivary secretion

   iii the skin becomes dry and inelastic

   iv the eyes appear sunken

   v eventual fall in blood pressure and pulse volume

   vi urinary output decreases, urinary concentration increases

   vii eventual constipation

   viii eventual temperature rise as evaporation of fluid from body surface decreases

   ix serum electrolyte imbalance

n i Protein is used in replacement in 'wear and tear' processes, for formation of new tissue as in periods of growth, during pregnancy and following injury for formation of substances which are protein in nature, e.g. enzymes, hormones, haemoglobin and plasma proteins.

   Protein is a source of energy — one gram providing approx. 4 kcal.

   ii Carbohydrate is oxidised in the body to give heat and energy for all forms of body activity. One gram providing 4 kcal.

   iii Fats form a part of cell structure.

   Fat depositions around internal organs help hold them in position and protects them from injury. Subcutaneous fat acts as an insulator. Assist in the absorption of fat-soluble vitamins from the intestine. Fats are oxidised in the body to provide heat and energy, each gram producing 9 kcal.

   iv Mineral salts are essential constituents of the soft tissues, fluids and skeleton and are necessary within the body for all body processes.

   v Vitamins which are a group of substances which exist in minute quantities in natural foods and are essential to normal nutrition especially for growth and development. They are divided into two main groups:

   Fat soluble   A.D.E. and K.

   Water soluble   B complex and C.

o   Discomfort affecting speech, oral infection, halitosis.
    Difficulty in swallowing, pharyngeal infection.
    Nausea, vomiting, loss of appetite, reluctance to drink, leading to
    further dehydration.
    Respiratory infection.

p   i   naso-gastric 'tube' feeding
    ii   gastrostomy 'tube' feeding
    iii intravenous
    iv   rectally

2 a Only 20 different amino acids are used in the formation of body
      protein. Of these, only eight are **essential amino acids** and must be
      present in the food protein. If they are present in the diet, the
      remaining twelve can be made by the liver.
   b First class protein is the term given to protein foods such as meat,
      fish, eggs, soya beans, which contain all the essential amino acids
      in the correct proportions.
   c The complex process whereby food which has been digested and
      absorbed is converted into heat and energy and used for growth
      and repair of tissues is termed **metabolism.**
      The build-up of complex materials from simpler components is
      known as **anabolism,** the breakdown of complex substances is
      known as **catabolism.**
   d Collections of lymphatic nodules in the distal portion of the small
      intestine which play an important part in the defence of the body
      against bacterial invasion, as in typhoid fever.
   e Refers to the movement by which the stomach and intestines propel
      their contents onwards. It consists of alternate waves of relaxation
      and contraction in succession along the tract.
   f Emaciation is a state of advanced wasting. It is associated with
      diseases of the alimentary system in which digestion is inefficient or
      in which food is not fully absorbed. It is a feature of advanced
      malignant disease, and may be a feature of a prolonged infectious
      process.
   g Cachexia refers to a state of general severe debility where the
      patient appears emaciated, very sick and feeble. It is seen in
      advanced disease states.
   h The maintenance of health depends upon the consumption and
      absorption of appropriate amounts of energy and all the nutrients.
      Too little or too much of some over a period of months may lead to
      malnutrition, e.g. **marasmus** in young children, **obesity, deficiency
      diseases:** scurvy, anaemias.
   i Loss of appetite.

j Enzymes are biological catalysts — they are proteins which accelerate the rate of a specific chemical reaction without themselves being affected. Enzymes break down the constituents of the food (as it passes along the digestive tract) into small molecules suitable for absorption into the blood.

k May be a symptom of oesophageal hernia. It results from incompetence of the cardiac sphincter allowing reflux of peptic juice into the lower oesophagus and may result in ulceration and inflammation.

l Comprises a regime of **i** gastric aspiration by means of nasogastric suction which helps to decompress the bowel and keep the stomach empty, and **ii** intravenous replacements of fluid and electrolytes.

m A state of atony of the intestine — where the normal peristaltic movements which propel the intestinal contents along are absent.

n The secretory cells in the small intestine which secrete intestinal juice (succus entericus).

o Spasm of the lower oesophagus. A neuromuscular failure of relaxation at the lower end of the oesophagus which may lead to progressive dilatation of the oesophagus above.

p A diagnostic test which requires the withdrawal of small amounts of gastric juice through a nasogastric tube at intervals for a period of one to two hours after gastric secretion has been stimulated, usually by an intramuscular injection of a substance such as histamine, pentagastrin or insulin.

3

a	iv or i	**e**	iv or i	**i**	v
b	vii	**f**	xii	**j**	viii
c	x	**g**	ii	**k**	vi
d	xi	**h**	iii	**l**	ix

9 HELPING THE PATIENT TO REST AND SLEEP

Being able to rest and being able to relax are not necessarily the same thing.

Being able to relax may involve activity which is enjoyed by the individual and which helps him to find freedom from stress, anxiety and the constraints and demands made upon him.

Rest usually refers to 'a state of repose', 'a cessation from motion or labour', in other words, rest refers to a state in which activity is markedly reduced.

The ways in which we relax and rest or the methods we use to achieve relaxation and rest have been developed to suit our individual needs and to fit into our life pattern. We may need to lie down alone in a quiet room in order to feel rested, we may be able to rest in a comfortable chair in a room full of people, or we may like to listen to soft music, or read a book before we can feel relaxed enough to rest for example. Generally speaking, if we are allowed to or able to relax and rest, we feel better as a result, we feel more able to cope with demands made upon us.

Sleep is a period of loss of consciousness from which we can be easily roused. The dictionary describes sleep as 'the condition normally recurrent every night and lasting some hours in which the eyes are closed and the nervous system inactive'. This simple explanation does not reflect the complex phenomenon that is sleep and a great deal of research is going on into **what it is, whether we need it, why we need it,** and **what happens if we are deprived of it**. The way in which we achieve sleep, like rest, varies with the individual; we develop habits in relation to **promoting sleep** and to **sleep patterns**, just as we develop habits in relation to other daily activities.

Each individual's sleep needs differ, but it is thought that the majority of individuals sleep for about 8 hours in 24, how much of this is due to a real **need** for sleep and how much is due to **conditioning** is not really clear.

Patients in hospital usually have their sleep habits/patterns altered, in fact it has been implied that patients themselves do not expect to sleep well in hospital, and many nurses are also of the opinion that patients cannot expect to sleep as well in hospital as they do at home. However, there is much that the nurse can do to help the patient to rest and to sleep once they are in hospital. Some of the measures are general and would apply to all patients, some are specific to the needs of particular patients.

Environmental factors

These are outside influences which may affect a patient's ability to sleep.
1 The size of the ward, the position of the bed in the ward, and the

presence of other people sleeping in the same room/ward. At home, most people either sleep alone or share a room with one other person.

2 The temperature/humidity in the ward, the nearness of the bed to hot radiators or draughty windows or doors. At home one might like to sleep near an open window, others might like a warm bedroom or they might have preferences as to where their bed should be in relation to the door, for example.

3 The noises in a hospital ward may be disturbing for the patient, they may be from other patients, e.g. snoring, groaning, restlessness; from equipment, e.g. electric fans or mattresses, oxygen and suction apparatus, monitors; from staff, e.g. nurses talking, telephones, clatter from the ward kitchen, doors banging, staff attending to a patient's needs during the night.

4 Lighting can also be disturbing to the patient, lights left on in a corridor for example or above a patient's bed for any reason, or from the nurse's station or office.

5 More immediate to the patient, the type of bed or mattress might be different to that which he is used to, patients may be used to single or double sized beds, a soft or hard mattress, a certain number of blankets or pillows; the close proximity of equipment such as bed cradles, splints, traction equipment may make change of position or adoption of the most comfortable position difficult or even impossible.

Physical factors

The **general condition** of the patient and the **nature of the treatment** he is undergoing. As mentioned above the patient could be receiving i.v. therapy, could be attached to a monitor, may need continuous oxygen or frequent suction therapy, or nursing attention might be of a frequent or continuous nature.

His position, of necessity, might be different to that which he normally adopts to sleep, he might be restricted by the nature of his disorder and the medical/nursing instructions regarding his position, e.g. lying flat due to back injury, sitting up due to breathing difficulty, lying to one side to promote drainage or he might be restricted by some form of traction or by drainage apparatus attached to the side of the bed.

Any discomfort he may be experiencing from any of the above factors, or from a wound or specific injury may be relieved by general change of the patient's position, careful positioning of limbs, adjustments to bed linen and pillows, adjustments to equipment and/or administration of pain relieving drugs.

He might feel hot and sticky — uncomfortable due to excessive sweating or restrictive bedwear. A light wash and change of bedwear can be most refreshing and relaxing.

The need to go to the toilet might cause discomfort, the patient might be reluctant to ask for a bedpan or commode in the night, afraid that he is a bother or might disturb other patients.

Thirst and/or hunger can also prevent a patient from sleeping and the latter is a factor that is not readily considered by the nurse. The last meal of the hospital day is usually taken about 6 p.m., the patient then has to wait until about 8 a.m. the next day for breakfast. If one adds to this the fact that the patient might not be eating very well, one can see that hunger might be a more common problem than many nurses think. A hot drink and a snack can often be quite easily prepared and might be greatly appreciated by the patient.

Psychological factors

A patient who is worried or even afraid, usually finds difficulty in sleeping; he might find that he cannot get off to sleep or that he wakes frequently throughout the night. His anxieties might be related to himself, his hospitalisation, his condition or nature of treatment. He might be concerned about the effects of his illness on his relatives, on the family/domestic/financial situation, and on his employment; on the other hand his anxieties might not be directly related to himself but to concern for a member of his family.

Quite often, in the loneliness of the night, like most other problems, these anxieties appear worse than they really are.

From the outset and initial assessment of the patient, the aim should be to identify any of these problems so that nursing intervention can be directed towards solving or alleviating them.

Whenever possible the patient should be informed about all aspects of his hospitalisation, why various examinations/procedures/treatments are necessary, what they entail, what his role should be and in what way their implementation and after effects/care will effect him. Reassurance should be given throughout.

Whenever possible, the patient and his relatives should be interviewed in order to see how the hospitalisation is affecting the family and whether problems can be solved by the family themselves or whether referral to other support services is advisable. They should be afforded every opportunity to discuss any worries and fears they might have. The nurse must remember that often a patient might not be able to recognise his own problems or might be trying to deny that they exist. If she feels she is out of her depth in relation to this, she must inform her seniors so that they can take appropriate action.

10   HELPING THE PATIENT
TO COPE WITH PAIN

Pain is said to be the most common symptom that causes a person to seek advice/help from a doctor or hospital; it is the symptom that conveys to the individual that there is something wrong with his or her body. However, the experience that we call pain is a purely subjective one, even though patients can be said to be suffering from the same disease process, and may be 'labelled' with the same diagnosis, their pain experience is a personal one, we each perceive and react to pain differently. Exactly what each patient feels to be pain, what is each patient's threshold, how each describes his pain and how each responds to pain will vary considerably. Differences in social, cultural and educational background, previous experience of pain, knowledge of the situation or factors causing the pain, the intensity and duration of pain, the general state of physical, mental and emotional well-being and attention from and attitude of those around, will all account for the variations in the individual response to pain.

The nurse will be aware of the current theories that aim to explain the mechanism of pain, the specificity theory, the pattern theory, and the gate control theory, but even a detailed knowledge of sensory pathways to the brain does not necessarily help the nurse to understand the 'experience of pain' or help her to help the patient to cope with his pain. **Pain is whatever the experiencing person says it is and exists whenever he says it does;** if the nurse remembers this, she will never dismiss the patient's pain, rather she will accept that there is always a need to help the patient cope with his pain and will take appropriate steps to do so.

The first important step is to **assess the patient's pain**. Information may be obtained from the **nurse's observations,** from **verbal and written reports** from other people and from **relatives,** this is objectively recorded. Most important; and because of the subjectivity of pain, the patient should be allowed whenever possible, **to describe or indicate what and how he feels in his own words**. However, it must be said at this point that the use of words as an indicator and measurement of pain is fraught with the danger of misunderstanding on the part of both the patient and the nurse. There are now various methods which aim to find a reliable way of measuring pain and range from stimulus devices, the pain thermometer, to pain scale indicator cards.

The following information can be obtained from the patient (subjective recording).

1 The location, type, intensity of the pain.
2 The time and type of onset and the duration of each episode.
3 Signs within the locality of pain.

4   The position or movements adopted by the patient.
5   The general appearance and the emotional response of the patient.
6   The existence of provoking or relieving factors.
7   The presence of associated symptoms.

If an underlying cause for the pain can be identified, medical intervention can be directed towards relieving the pain; this might take the form of a surgical procedure, a manipulative procedure, an immobilisation procedure or a pressure relieving procedure, or might involve the administration of drugs which directly or indirectly bring the patient relief.

Sometimes a multi-disciplinary approach to pain relief may be adopted, i.e. together with medical and nursing intervention, the patient will be referred to the physiotherapy department for pain relieving measures such as passive or active exercises, specific mobilisation programmes, manipulative or specific therapy (heat, electrical stimulation).

Nursing measures to relieve pain

Although it is the doctor who prescribes the analgesia, the nurse should not think of its administration as the first or only measure to be used to relieve pain. On the other hand, analgesia should never be withheld when its use is necessary. Analgesia therefore is used alongside other nursing measures in order to provide pain relief.

Physical measures

a   **Helping the patient to achieve maximum comfort** by correct positioning, change of position, adjustments and changes of bedlinen, bedwear and pillows, attention to wounds, change of dressings, care of drainage tubes etc.
b   **Helping the patient to rest/relax** by planning care and analgesic regime to allow for adequate rest periods, the use of pillows, splints etc., to support, immobilise or alleviate a painful area and teaching the patient how to relax by deep breathing and other muscle group exercises.
c   **Providing stimulation which interferes with or blocks pain transmission.** This includes measures such as massage, local counter-irritants, e.g. menthol, heat application and electrical stimulation.

Psychological measures include:

Helping the patient to be less anxious about the pain by being available to discuss **any** problems that the patient may have and by offering appropriate help; by teaching the patient about anticipated pain and the events surrounding the pain, e.g. when to expect pain, the type of pain and the measures that can be taken to relieve the pain; by discussing with the patient why his particular pain occurs and the meaning of pain in terms that he will understand; by providing distraction which will reduce his concentration on his pain, for example, acceptable sensory stimulation such as radio, T.V., conversation, visitors; by giving appropriate supportive and symptomatic care whilst the patient is experiencing his pain.

Analgesia

As mentioned earlier, it is the doctor who prescribes the medication used for pain relief, the nurse gives the drugs according to the doctor's orders; however, the instructions may allow for the use of discretion on the nurse's part, i.e. analgesics may be prescribed 'prn' or 'if necessary 4–6 hrly'. This means that control of a patient's pain is very much a nursing responsibility.

Analgesics can broadly be divided into two categories:

Narcotic analgesics e.g. morphine, usually used for the relief of severe pain, these work by acting on the central nervous system and one of the most undesirable side-effects is dependency.

Non-narcotic analgesics e.g. aspirin, used widely for the relief of less severe pain and which work by acting on the peripheral nerves at the site of the pain and of which the most undesirable side effects are due to toxicity.

The best pain relief medication is that which provides the greatest relief from pain with the least number of undesirable side effects or complications. Nursing responsibilities therefore include:

1 Adequate assessment and observation of the patient in order that recognition of pain can be prompt and appropriate pain-relieving measures can be taken.

2 Knowledge of analgesic drugs, their properties, their mode of action, the desirable and undesirable patient responses and the alternatives that can best be used in combination with other medication.

When pain cannot be relieved by the more common methods, nerve blocks using local anaesthetic drugs or surgical interruption of nerve pathways may be considered necessary. In recent years, the use of acupuncture, hypnotherapy and psychoprophylaxis as supplements to or alternatives to the more traditional methods of pain relief have increased. The growth of Pain Relief Clinics and the increased awareness of a more positive approach to pain relief for those patients with protracted pain have led to a new dimension in nursing. Rather than simply carrying out medical orders relating to pain relief, nurses are now taking on a more important role with regard to assessment and subsequent treatment of the patient and are beginning to 'specialise' in this field of care.

Practice Questions
1 Answer the following questions
a What is a pain receptor?

b List the information you would obtain from the patient who is complaining of pain.

c What observations would you make on the lower arm of a patient who has sustained an injury to his elbow and is complaining of numbness of hand?

d Give an example of a narcotic drug; briefly describe how narcotics work.

e What are the most common undesirable side-effects of morphine?

f What signs/symptoms might lead you to suspect that a newly applied plaster of paris (below knee) is too tight?

g What are the four cardinal signs of inflammation? Explain briefly how they occur.

h Differentiate between dyspnoea and orthopnoea.

i List the measures (other than the administration of analgesia) which may help relieve a patient's pain.

j Differentiate between analgesia and anaesthesia.

2 What do you understand by the following terms
a Pain threshold

b Referred pain

c Phantom pain

d Intractable pain

e Abdominal guarding

f Cardiogenic shock

g Colic

h Strangury

i Dysuria

j Tenesmus

k Heartburn

l Neuralgia

m Intermittent claudication.

n Migraine

o Ischaemia

Answers
1

a Pain receptors are the freely branching bare nerve endings which form a diffuse network in the skin, on joint surfaces, in deep tissue and viscera. From the pain receptor the stimuli passes along different nerve fibres into the spinal cord or brain stem and on to the sensory cortex of the brain.

b The type of pain, e.g. burning, aching, throbbing, stabbing, the location — as exact as possible, e.g. frontal, temporal, umbilical, whether localised or diffuse, the intensity and duration of the pain, e.g. severe, intermittent, the type of onset, e.g. gradual, sudden. The position adopted by the ptient, e.g. lying still, rolling about, presence of signs at the site of the pain, e.g. swelling, tenderness, the general appearance and emotional response of the patient, the existence of provoking or relieving factors, the presence of associated symptoms, the vital signs, temperature, pulse, respiratory and blood pressure levels.

c There may be arterial injury, particularly if there is a supracondylar fracture. The nurse should be particularly observant for, and frequently note any changes in

pain
pallor including temperature
pulse or absence of pulse
paraesthesia
paralysis
Comparison should be made with the other hand and arm.

d The most widely known narcotic drug is probably **morphia**. Narcotic analgesics work by depressing the central nervous system, e.g. morphia acts on the periaqueductal grey matter of the brain, thus relieving pain; other sensory perceptions are less affected.

e Respiratory depression, nausea and vomiting, euphoria or dysphoria, tolerance to and dependence on the narcotic drug, constipation.

f Swelling, blueness, coldness, pallor, prolonged blanching, numbness, pins and needles and difficulty in moving the toes. Pain anywhere under the plaster, at the plaster edges, or in the toes.

g Redness, heat, swelling, pain.
Redness and heat — due to local vaso-dilatation, increased local blood supply and slowing of blood flow through the affected area.
Swelling — Histamine and other chemicals are released by the injured tissue cells, causing increased permeability of the blood vessel walls. This, together with the increased filtration pressure, allows plasma and blood cells particularly leukocytes to pass out into the interstitial spaces.
Pain — the increased interstitial volume causes pressure on the bare nerve endings.

h Dyspnoea describes a difficulty in breathing experienced by the patient; it is a subjective awareness of a disturbance in breathing.
Orthopnoea is dyspnoea which is present when the patient is lying down but is appreciably relieved by elevation of the trunk.

i **Achieving maximum comfort**
Correct positioning and/or adjustments to the patient's position.

E

Adjustments to clothing or bedlinen which will make patient more comfortable.

Attention to wound dressings, drainage apparatus, etc.

Achieving rest/relaxation

Planning care to allow for rest periods, teaching patients how to relax all or parts of body by means of muscle group exercises and positioning.

Adequate support to all or parts of the body.

Bathing, massage, measures requested by the patient and not contra-indicated by his condition.

Providing information which will help relieve anxiety

Discussion and help with problems, talking to the patient about his pain, what to expect, how it will be relieved.

Providing diversion or distraction from the pain

Any sensory stimulation that is acceptable to the patient and not contra-indicated by his illness.

Providing supportive care

Being with the patient, holding his hand, bathing his face, adjusting his pillows etc.

j Analgesics relieve pain without loss of consciousness; they may depress pain perception, reduce the patient's response to pain, or relax muscle spasm.

Anaesthesia means loss of the power of feeling. It can be applied to loss over a limited area of skin produced by certain nervous diseases, by freezing or by local anaesthetic drugs or to a total loss of feeling and consciousness as achieved by general anaesthesia.

2

a Pain threshold — the point at which awareness of pain takes place. It can be alleviated by distraction, stimuli from other parts of the body and by events which depress the activity of the cerebral cortex, e.g. drugs, alcohol, shock. It can be lowered by injury or inflammation of the parts involved with the pain sensation and by reduction of other stimuli.

b Pain originating in an organ but felt elsewhere, e.g. internal organs derive their nervous control from the sympathetic nervous system through which they often obtain complicated and very distant connections with the brain and spinal cord. Pain in an organ is often referred, in what seems at first sight to be a bizarre manner, to distant points.

c This refers to the sensation of pain felt in a limb that is no longer there. If a nerve is stimulated by pressure at some point along its route, the sensation felt is usually assumed to be coming from the receptor at the distal end. Stimulation of the cut ends of the nerves following amputation gives rise to the sensation of a phantom limb. It may take a long time for the body image to be modified.

d Intractable pain refers to prolonged pain which often cannot be effectively controlled by analgesics. Unlike acute pain it might not be possible to predict when it will end.

e Rigidity developing in the abdominal muscles may be associated with rebound tenderness and elicited by abdominal palpation.

f Shock describes a clinical state of pallor, sweating, coldness, peripheral cyanosis, rapid weak pulse and low blood pressure, resulting from inadequate tissue and organ perfusion. Cardiogenic shock indicates an inadequate cardiac output and is associated with cardiac conditions.

g Colic refers to severe spasmodic pain usually arising from the presence of a substance within a tubular structure which excites spasmodic contraction of the muscular coats of the tube, e.g. biliary colic, renal colic.

h Strangury describes the condition in which there is a constant desire to pass water, accompanied by a straining sensation, though only a few drops, often blood stained, can be voided.

i Dysuria — difficulty or pain in urinating.

j Tenesmus describes a constant full feeling in the rectum and the desire to defaecate together with straining at stool and the passage of little but mucus and sometimes blood.

k Heartburn is felt as a burning sensation experienced in the region of the heart, sometimes up into the back of the throat or behind the sternum and is usually caused by irritation of the oesophageal mucosa by reflux of gastric acid fluid from the stomach.

l Neuralgia literally means nerve pain and means the existence of pain in some portion of, or throughout the whole of, the distribution of a sensory nerve.

m Intermittent claudication is characterised by pain in the legs (particularly the calves) after walking a certain distance. The pain is relieved by resting for a short time. It is due to arteriosclerosis of the arteries to the leg, which results in inadequate blood supply to the muscles particularly noticed during exercise.

n Migraine is a condition characterised by a recurring intense headache; in susceptible individuals it can be provoked by a wide variety of factors and the headache can take a number of forms.

o Ischaemia describes a deficient blood supply to an organ or tissue, usually as a result of contraction, spasm, constriction or blockage of the arteries supplying that part.

11 HELPING THE PATIENT TO AVOID HAZARDS IN THE ENVIRONMENT

Florence Nightingale once said 'the hospital should do the patient no harm'.

When a person is healthy, he tries to organise his life, within certain constraints, to suit himself. As far as he is able, he will try to exercise at least some control over the events that make up his life pattern. Consequently, and often for his own and his family's convenience, he develops a habitual pattern to his daily living activities, he chooses whether to promote health in himself and his family and he takes necessary steps to protect himself and his family from danger inside and outside his home.

When a person becomes a patient in hospital, his daily life pattern obviously changes, but in addition he tends to lose control of the organisational aspects of certain activities and he has to depend on others to a much larger extent than previously to ensure his safety/well-being.

Hazards associated with being in hospital
Loss of independence

There have been frequent references throughout this book to the maintenance or improvement of the patient's level of independence. Nurses often, through kindness, sometimes for convenience to themselves as well as the patient, but usually not as a result of assessment of the patient's needs, do too much for their patients. On a short term basis this might do very little harm, the patient may feel that is is rather nice to be 'spoiled', to have everything done for them, but for many patients and certainly those with long-term illness, allowing them to become nurse-institution dependent may not be in their best interest.

Nursing care should be based on the needs of each individual and incorporated in the nursing plan should be maximum use of the patient's self-care potential. In this way the patient is helped to keep his self-respect and dignity; involvement in the achievement of personal goals allows a sense of purpose to develop in those patients who would normally take a more passive role in their care; utilising the patient's self care ability begins the rehabilitative process at the earliest possible stage and, when complete recovery cannot be achieved, promoting the highest level of independence improves the quality of the patient's life.

Mistaken identity

Under normal circumstances, the individual is capable of and responsible enough to identify himself to others whenever it becomes necessary. He can correct the error if he is addressed by the wrong name or title, or if he is in receipt of anything which is not meant for him but someone else. Errors arising from mistaken identity are less likely to occur when individuals are capable of, have control of, and are responsible for identifying themselves. Unfortunately, under certain circumstance when patients are in hospital, such control and responsibility is partially or completely taken away from them. When the patient is very young, confused or unconscious, such a situation is understandable. However, similar situations occur when the nursing staff are responsible for the administration of drugs to patients, for preparing and delivering the correct patient for operation, for getting the correct patient to a particular department for investigation or treatment, for example. Although some patients may question events in hospital as they happen and will make queries if they have any doubts, many patients do not see themselves as responsible and tend to 'leave everything to the nurse'.

It is to minimize the risk of mistaken identity, that hospitals formulate policies and checking procedures for its staff (and patients) to follow — hence the current practice of using identity bracelets — but it usually follows that within guidelines laid down by employing authorities, it is usually the responsibility of the nurse/doctor to establish the identity of the patient by the most appropriate means available before proceeding to treatment.

Infection

Hospitals carry a high risk of infection. The source of the infection may be the hospital environment itself, a variety of pathogenic organisms may be found in greater concentrations and may be of virulent and antibiotic-resistant strains, it may be the staff within the hospital or the source may be the patients themselves. One of the particular dangers of being a patient in hospital is that of infection passing from one patient to another. The patients most at risk are those at either end of the age range, the very young and the elderly, those with chronic and debilitating diseases, those receiving therapy which lowers the patient's resistance to infection, e.g. immunosuppressive, steroid or cytotoxic drugs, radiotherapy and patients with extensive skin loss.

Together with this knowledge, the nurse should remember that all entry procedures carry the risk of introducing infection into the body, e.g. cutting operations, all forms of catheterization, intubation, injections venepunctures and intravenous therapy, to mention a few.

The effects of such hospital-acquired infections can be considered from a number of points of view.

a   The immediate effects of pain, discomfort anxiety to the patient and his relatives.

b   The additional treatment required to counteract the effects of the infection which may range between additional rest, drug therapy, and surgical intervention and which may mean a prolonged stay in hospital.

c The additional nursing and medical time involved in treating the patient.

d The longer-term effects which might mean a more lengthy rehabilitative period, or even permanent disability affecting the quality of life or even decreasing life expectancy.

e The considerable additional cost of the extended hospital stay both to the hospital (cost per in-patient week) and to the patient and his relatives (visiting costs, loss of earning power), and the unavailability of the hospital bed to anyone else.

Every nurse should be aware of the relentless efforts that should be made by all relevant hospital personnel to prevent and combat the spread of infection within the hospital. This means that everyone should adhere to basic rules of personal and hospital hygiene, everyone should follow the safe codes of practice that apply to hospital procedures, and all relevant personnel should be aware of and adhere to the principles of asepsis whenever necessary.

The aims of care related to hospital-acquired infection are as follows.

a Increasing the resistance of the patient to infection by improving and supporting his own defence mechanisms.

b Destruction of the organism causing the disease.

c Providing the necessary care required by the patient in order to combat the effects of, and provide relief from, the infective process.

d Prevention of the spread of infection to others.

Most hospitals now have Control of Infection Committees and Control of Infection Officers whose responsibility it is to monitor the incidence of infection in their areas and make appropriate recommendations for improvement.

Drug therapy

In hospital the administration of drugs is usually the responsibility of the nursing staff. The doctor prescribes the drug therapy, the pharmacist makes available drugs to the ward staff and the nursing staff follow the medical instructions as to **how much** of **which** drug will be given to **which patient** by **what route** and **when**.

Patients do not normally have very much knowledge about the drugs they are receiving, of the desirable and undesirable effects, nor about the combined effects of drugs, other than the information the doctor, pharmacist, or nurse have deemed it necessary for him to know.

Whilst he is in hospital the safety of the patient with regard to drug therapy is often in the hands of others. When he goes home the responsibility becomes his own or his relatives, perhaps with assistance from the primary health care team.

Iatrogenic disease (disease caused by treatment)
It is now recognised and accepted that as a result of drug toxicity, a wide variety of disorders may arise as a side-effect of drug treatment, particularly when a combination of drugs is prescribed for one patient. Such reactions may be dose-related or non dose-related and may occur with all age groups. However, the elderly patient is particularly susceptible because of the combined effect of the variety of drugs they may be taking, because of cumulation of drugs as a result of impaired renal function, and because of non-adherence to their drug schedule at home for whatever reasons.

The responsibility of the nurse therefore includes seeing that:

i   each patient receives the correct dose of the correct drugs at the correct time by the correct route.

ii the ordering, transport, storage, safety and administration of all drugs at ward level adheres to the statutory and local regulations and policies.

iii she is aware of the normal dosage range, desired patient response and undesirable patient responses that might be expected from the common drugs or combination of drugs in use.

iv she is aware of where to obtain necessary information/instruction related to drug therapy.

v   wherever necessary the patient and/or his relatives are appropriately informed about the particular drug he is receiving and are appropriately instructed regarding their participation in the therapy.

Health and safety
When a person is healthy, he is able to protect himself from the dangers around him. He is usually able and responsible enough to recognise danger and then take what he considers are the necessary measures. These measures might result in a change of response in the individual or adaptations to his environment.

When a person becomes ill, he may become unable to cope with this responsibility and he then becomes dependent on others to protect him from danger. When the person is admitted to hospital, the responsibility is partially and sometimes totally transferred to the hospital staff. They may then have to protect the patient and his relatives from the dangers that arise from being in hospital.

In almost every ward and department of a hospital there are potential hazards. The purpose of the Health and Safety at Work Act 1974, is to provide a framework to encourage high standards of health and safety in the workplace, thus eliminating or minimising the risk to the health and safety of the individuals therein. The aim of the Act is to involve everyone, management and all personnel, and to make everyone aware of the importance of Health and Safety. Employees have a duty under the

Act to take reasonable care to avoid injury to themselves or to others by their work activities and to co-operate with employers in meeting statutory requirements. It is clear that the nursing staff, by nature of their close involvement with patients, have particular responsibilities in this field, thus every nurse, by virtue of their knowledge and training should be able to:

i   recognise what constitutes a hazard and deal with it effectively, either by direct action or by reporting the hazard to others better equipped/qualified to deal with it.

ii adhere to all safe codes of practice (for example, those dealing with fire, explosion, radiation and care and custody of drugs), and take the necessary course of action should an emergency situation arise.

Practice Questions

1 Answer the following questions

a What are exteroceptors?

b List the protective functions of the skin.

c Differentiate in list form between surface and inner defence mechanisms.

d Explain briefly the events that occur in a reflex action.

e Differentiate between primary, reactionary and secondary haemorrhage.

f List the **local** complications that might occur following abdominal surgery (in the first three weeks).

g How would you position an unconscious patient and why?

h What colour is an oxygen cylinder?

i List the immediate checks that would be made before a patient leaves the ward for the operating theatre.

j What are the common sites used for intramuscular injection?

k List the hazards associated with the administration of oxygen.

l Differentiate between source and protective isolation.

m What signs/symptoms might lead you to suspect a wound infection?

n What precautions are taken to ensure that the correct patient receives the correct drug?

o What might be the significance of a 'swinging' temperature following surgery?

p Differentiate between active and passive immunity.

q List the hazards of prolonged bedrest.

r What specific information should be elicited from a woman of child-bearing age prior to abdominal/pelvic X-ray?

s What signs/symptoms would lead you to suspect a mismatched blood transfusion?

t Differentiate between sterilization and disinfection.

2 What do you understand by the following terms

a Pre-operative bowel preparation

b Controlled drug

c Notifiable disease

d Pathogenic organism

e Agranulocytosis

f Retrolental fibroplasia

g Pseudomonas pyocyanae

h Incubation period

i Monoamine oxidase inhibitors

j Bacteraemic shock

k Concussion

l Sub-clinical attack

m Wound dihesence
n Pulmonary embolism
o Iatrogenic disease

Answers
1
a Sensory nerve endings which sense stimuli from outside the body.
b The continuity of the skin, its ability to rapidly heal itself following injury and the bacteriostatic agents secreted in the sebum protects the internal structures from injury, drying and the invasion of organisms. The production of the pigment melanin helps protect the body from damaging doses of ultra-violet light.

The presence of sensory receptors and nerves in the skin serve as a protective mechanism for the body as well as conveying impulses that contribute information about the external environment.

It is also protective in that, by altering the calibre of its blood vessels and by activating sweat glands, it plays an important role in body temperature regulation.
c **Surface defences**
  i Skin
  ii Mucous membranes
  iii Secretions, e.g. tears
              gastric juice
              respiratory mucus
  iv Mechanical arrangement of structures, e.g. respiratory passages, ciliated epithelium, length of male urethra compared to female
Inner defences
Phagocytosis
Bacteriolysis
Inflammatory response
Immune response
d A reflex action is one of the simplest forms of activity of the nervous system.

A sensory receptor is stimulated — the impulse travels along the sensory pathway to the spinal cord — within the spinal cord the impulse passes through a synaptic contact to a motor cell which passes the impulse down the motor pathway and a muscular contraction results. A simple example of reflex action is given by the drawing away of the hand when it is pricked with a pin, before and independently of the conscious perception of pain.
e i Primary — at the time of injury, operation, event.
  ii Reactionary — usually within the first 24 hours when the blood pressure returns to normal.
  iii Secondary — after 5–7 days because of erosion of a blood vessel by infection or malignant disease.

f Reactionary haemorrhage
  Paralytic ileus
  Infection of wound
  Peritonitis
  Abscess formation
  Secondary haemorrhage
  Anastamotic or wound breakdown
  Formation of adhesions.

g The first priority is the establishment of a patent airway. He should be placed in a lateral or semi-prone position (unless contra-indicated by chest or spinal injury) with the neck in line with the spine, possibly with the bed in a slight head down tilt. This allows drainage of mucus or vomit and prevents obstruction of the airway by the tongue. If either of these two positions is not possible and the patient has to be nursed in the dorsal position, an artificial airway may be needed.

h Black with a white shoulder.

i Identity — correct patient for correct operation.
  Preparation has been completed, e.g.
      skin — shaved, cleansed,
      marked if necessary
      bladder emptied
      temperature recorded
      premedication given
      consent form signed
  Specific preparation related to operation, e.g. insertion of naso-gastric tube, catheterization.
  All notes, X-rays, investigative reports are available.

j Lateral-medial aspect of middle third of thigh (the belly of the vastus lateralis muscle).
  Antero-lateral aspect of middle third of thigh (the belly of the rectus femoris).
  Upper-outer quadrant of buttock (gluteal muscles).
  Upper-outer aspect of upper arm (the belly of the deltoid muscle).

k Explosion, fire, under-administration due to faulty apparatus, inadequate supervision, discontinuity of oxygen flow, over-administration in certain pulmonary diseases leading to respiratory depression or in the case of babies, too high a concentration leading to retrolental fibroplasia.
  Drying of the mucous membranes.

l Source isolation — the patient is isolated because he has an infection. He will be barrier nursed to prevent infection spreading from him to others.
  Protective isolation — the patient is isolated because he has a condition which makes him very susceptible to infection. He will be

reverse barrier nursed to prevent infection from others from spreading to him.

m Pyrexia — low grade, medium – high or intermittant.

Itching, dampness, tenderness under wound dressing, swelling/inflammation of wound. Discharge from wound.

n Name of the drug, dosage, time to be administered and route of administration are checked on the prescription sheet, the prescription should carry the doctor's signature. The identity of the patient is checked with identification details on the prescription sheet. The details on the prescription sheet are checked with the information label or the drug container. Many hospitals follow the rule that all drugs administration should be checked by a second nurse.

o It might be significant of a deep-seated infection — a collection of pus.

p Active immunity may be naturally or artificially acquired and involves the individual making his own antibodies in response to the stimulus of an antigen. This immunity develops slowly, persists for a long time and is associated with long-lasting specific reactivity of the antibody-forming tissues.

Passive immunity may be naturally or artificially acquired and involves the individual **receiving** ready-made antibodies from another person or animal. Immunity is rapidly established but is of shorter duration than above. There is no education of the antibody-forming tissues and therefore no potential immunity.

q Loss of interest, boredom, depression.

Loss of appetite — eventual loss of weight — constipation.

Shallow breathing — eventual chest infection.

Inadequate fluid intake — inadequate mobility — stones in kidney.

Stagnation of urine in bladder — infection (urinary tract).

Pressure sores.

Deep vein thrombosis. Pulmonary embolus.

Joint stiffne..s, muscle wasting, foot drop, osteoporosis.

r The date of her last period — to elicit the possibility of early stages of pregnancy.

s Pyrexia, headache, anxiety, restlessness.

Rigor/chill.

Backache (pain in the loin).

Chest pain (difficulty in breathing), tachycardia, palpitation.

Anaphylactic shock may develop — blood pressure falls, skin becomes cold and clammy, pulse is weak, patient may be disorientated/drowsy.

t **Sterilization** — the complete removal or destruction of all micro-organisms including the most resistant bacterial spores.

Disinfection — the removal or destruction of non-sporing vegetative organisms to varying degrees. Bacterial spores are not usually destroyed by disinfection processes.

2 May be

a requested prior to intestinal surgery and usually involves a combination of fluid diet, 'sterilization' of the bowel by oral antimicrobial drugs to destroy intestinal organisms (e.g. phthalylsulfathiazole, necrimycin) and possibly mechanical preparation (e.g. rectal washouts) of the bowel over a period of 3-4 days before operation.

b These are drugs, the use of which are covered by *The Misuse of Drugs Act 1971*, which is concerned with the control of narcotic drugs and other substances which can cause drug dependence. The Act gives a schedule of controlled drugs which includes all the substances previously covered by the *Dangerous Drugs Act*.

c Notifiable diseases are those, usually of an infectious nature, which are required by law to be made known to a health officer or local authority, e.g. anthrax, cholera, food poisoning, measles, meningitis.

d An organism capable of causing disease.

e A condition in which the granular variety of the white cells, is greatly reduced, thus markedly reducing the invidivual's resistance to infection. It may arise as a result of i. the toxic effects of certain drugs, ii. certain diseases e.g. typhoid, miliary tubercolosis, or iii. severe infections.

f A disturbance of the retina which was responsible for a high proportion of blindness in children, due to the administration of excessive amounts of oxygen to premature infants.

g A micro-organism found occasionally in the faeces of a normal person, rarely found in air or dust, but which finds liquid a congenial habitat. It is one of the bacterial organisms most frequently involved in hospital acquired infections. Infections due to Ps. pyocyanea have increased both in number and severity in the last 20 years.

h The period between invasion of body by a micro-organism and the clinical manifestations of an infection and during which the organisms are multiplying.

i These are drugs which are used for the treatment of depressive states and which destroy or prevent the action of a naturally occurring enzyme in the body (monoamine oxidase) which is concerned with the breakdown of monoamines. An excessive accumulation of monoamines can induce a dangerous reaction in the patient. Patients who are receiving these drugs are not allowed to eat foodstuffs containing tyramine (e.g. cheese, marmite, tinned fish).

j The clinical state of shock due to an overwhelming infection most often caused by gram-negative organisms. These release an endotoxin which causes eventual vasodilation and pooling of blood. The toxaemia may have a depressant cardiac action.

k Concussion refers to a violent jarring of the brain or spinal cord as a result of injury and is characterised by a short period of unconsciousness, pallor, pulse rate and respirations depressed; the patient may be dazed, confused, restless and unable to recall what has happened. There may be vomiting and headache. There is usually spontaneous recovery.

l An infection in which the signs are so mild that a diagnosis is not made and the patient may be unaware that he has had the disease.

m Wound breakdown (burst wound).

n The condition in which material (e.g. clot) has been carried through the blood vessels, often from the veins of the lower abdomen or legs to the pulmonary vessels where it has become lodged. The severity depends upon the size of the clot. It may be characterised by sudden chest pain, breathlessness, haemoptysis, shock; if large enough it may prove immediately fatal.

o Disease caused by treatment.

12 HELPING THE PATIENT
   WITH PROBLEMS OF MOBILITY

There are various ways of looking at the needs of an individual but whether one considers them from a daily living activity basis or from a hierarchical viewpoint, each individual's ability to satisfy his needs is very closely related to his ability to move.

It is only when one's range of movements becomes restricted, that one realises how much it affects one's lifestyle. Each patient's level of dependency is closely related to his degree of mobility and quite clearly, as a result of restrictions in mobility, there is difficulty or inability to carry out other activities such as washing, eating, breathing, eliminating etc. On a higher level, one's ability to socialise as one wants, pursue recreational activities, carry on employment, pursue a chosen career, fulfill personal ambitions may also be affected.

Purposeful movement involves the co-ordinated activity of the skeletal system, the muscular system and the nervous system and disturbance of these systems at any level may ultimately result in impaired mobility.

The aims of nursing care related to the mobility disturbance can therefore be seen as giving assistance appropriate to the degree/extent of impaired mobility in order to:

1 promote comfort and rest
2 promote optimal activity and exercise
3 maintain or improve the level of dependency
4 prevent and correct deformities
5 prevent complications that result from restricted mobility.

The first important principle is to define exactly what the patient's mobility disturbance is.

Consider the following examples:

		Treatment
Mr. A	Age 70 years broken Femur	Application of Thomas's
Mrs. B	Age 55 years broken Femur	Splint with Balanced
Mr. C	Age 20 years broken Femur	Traction
Master D	Age 6 years broken Femur	

It is true that as a result of the type of treatment prescribed, all four patients may spend some time confined to bed, but there the similarity might end; their individual differences will determine their specific mobility disturbance.

For example:

Apart from his fractured femur, Mr. C is a fit, energetic, athletic, young man who is able to lift himself, move around in bed and is able and willing to perform active limb exercises.

Mrs. B is obese, arthritic and unable to lift herself using the over-head hoist because of stiffness of shoulder joints and weak hand-grip.

Mr. A, a frail 70 year old, is able to move around in bed but is reluctant to do so and needs maximum encouragement.

Master D, well; anyone who has worked on a children's ward will know that, apart from, or perhaps despite being, 'tied to the bed' Master D's range of movement appears at times to be so unrestricted that there is very little he is unable to do.

As can be seen, in determining the degree of restriction, the nurse has, at the same time assessed the patient's self-care ability. Help towards coping with the mobility disturbance can then be planned specifically to meet the patient's needs.

In planning the nursing activities appropriate to the stated goal(s) for each patient, the nurse may consider the following:

When the patient is confined to bed

1   The aids/equipment that may be used to position the patient,
  a   comfortably and correctly
  b   to prevent and correct deformity
  c   to prevent the complications of restricted mobility e.g. pillows, special mattresses, foam pieces, sheepskin pieces, splints, backrests, limb rests.
2   The aids that are most appropriate to the patient's particular mobility disturbance and which would promote mobility e.g. use of overhead hoist, use of pulleys attached to bed frame, use of cotside or frame attached to bedside.
3   The explanation/instruction that can be given to the patient in order to encourage him to carry out active exercises and his own mobility programme.

Much emphasis has been placed on **proper positioning** of the patient who is confined to bed. This is primarily a nursing responsibility, although occasionally specific instructions may be given by the medical staff.

Correct positioning appropriate to the specific condition of the patient may be aimed at:

a   maintaining an airway/helping the patient to breathe
b   maintenance of circulation to vital centres
c   ensuring maximum comfort
d   preventing contractures and the development of deformities
e   promoting drainage
f   resting a particular part of the body
g   preparation for a specific procedure to be performed

Changes of position which may be general or specific to a part of the body and which may be passively or actively achieved to:

a   prevent joint stiffness

b maintain muscle tone
c stimulate circulation
d prevent pressure sores
e help prevent pulmonary complications
f help prevent urinary stasis.

When the patient is not confined to bed and ambulancy and independency is being encouraged.

Appropriate choice of and instruction in using mobility aids, walking frames, tripods, sticks, crutches etc., will encourage confidence in the patient who needs to use them.

Use of adjustable height beds and supportive chairs positioned at the bedside will promote ambulancy in the patient who is being encouraged to mobilise unaided.

Chairs or stools positioned strategically between the bed and bathroom/toilet/dayroom areas will help the patient who can only walk so far without a rest.

Provision of a suitable chair, a suitable surface on which to put necessary toilet requisites and sensibly placed mirrors will allow the seated as well as the standing patient to wash themselves and attend to hair, make-up etc., unaided.

Advice regarding the wearing of sensible footwear and clothing instead of slippers and loose bedwear might improve the patient's stance, his sense of balance and his vision of the floor and his foot movements.

As can be seen by all the examples above, patient independence is paramount, his self-care ability is used to the full. The nurse should give whatever assistance is necessary, whenever it is necessary but always with the above points in mind.

You may require lecture notes and other revision texts to answer the following questions.

Practice Questions

Answer the following:
a Name and give the number of bones in the vertebral column.
b Distinguish between the primary and secondary curves of the vertebral column.
c Movements between individual bones of the vertebral column are limited; however, what are the movements of the column as a whole?
d Name the first two cervical bones.
e What particular movements does the shape and arrangement of these two bones allow?
f How are joints classified? Give examples of each.
g Synovial joints are further classified according to their range of movement. What are they?
h Name the three types of muscle.
i What are the highly developed properties of muscle tissue?
j What are the functions of skeletal muscle?
k Describe briefly the attachment of skeletal muscle.
l What is the neuromuscular junction?
m Describe the activity at the neuromuscular junction.
n What is muscle tone?
o What is an anterior horn?
p What is a motor unit?
q Differentiate between isotonic and isometric contraction.
r Where is the sensory cortex situated?
s What is an afferent nerve?
t What is a reflex action?

2 What do you understand by the following terms:
a Paralysis
b Upper motor neurone lesion
c Lower motor neurone lesion
d Apraxia
e Proprioception
f Optimum positioning of limbs
g Foot drop
h Active physiotherapy
i Passive physiotherapy
j Osteoporosis
k Muscle atrophy
l Deep vein thrombosis
m Muscular dystrophy
n Parasthaesia

3 Match the conditions/procedures in a–n to the positions listed in i–xiv

a Unconscious patient
b Pulmonary oedema
c Above knee amputation
d Immediate post-tonsillectomy
e Dyspnoea due to lt. sided fractured ribs
f Cardiac arrest
g Post bilateral stripping of varicose veins
h Post operative shock
i Lower lumbar injury
j Lumbar puncture
k Abdominal paracentesis
l Administration of enema
m Taking a high vaginal swab
n Rectal washout

   i Left lateral
  ii Left lateral
 iii Sims
 iv Recumbent on firm base
  v Lateral spine fully flexed
 vi Sitting upright
vii Semi-recumbent with periods in prone position
viii Foot of bed elevated
 ix Sitting — inclined to left side
  x Recumbent
 xi Semi-prone
 xii Recumbent – head down tilt
xiii Semi-prone
xiv Semi-recumbent

Answers
1a The vertebral column consists of:
    24 separate and irregular bones
        7 cervical
        12 thoracic
        5 lumbar
    and 9 fused bones
        5 sacral
        4 coccygeal
b The thoracic and sacral primary curves are concave anteriorly.
The cervical and lumbar secondary curves are convex anteriorly.

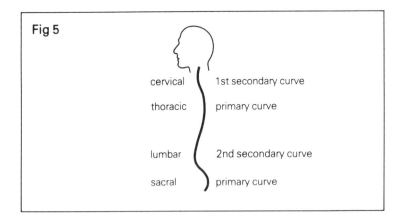

Fig 5

cervical — 1st secondary curve
thoracic — primary curve
lumbar — 2nd secondary curve
sacral — primary curve

c Flexion — bending forward
Extension — bending backward
Lateral flexion — bending to the side
Rotation — turning round
d i Atlas
    ii Axis
e The two articular facets of the atlas form joints with the condyles of the occipital bone of the skull allowing **nodding movement of the head.**
The odontoid process of the axis articulates with the first cervical vertebra allowing **rotation of the head.**
f Joints are classified according to the amount of movement possible between the articulating surfaces.
Fixed joints where **no movement** is possible, e.g. bones of the skull.
Slightly moveable joints where there is a pad of cartilage between the

bone surfaces allowing **slight movement,** e.g. symphysis pubis vertebral column.

Freely moveable joints or **synovial** joints, e.g. shoulder, hip, wrist, knee.

g **Hinge** joints — flexion and extension only, e.g. elbow, knee.

Gliding joints — articular surfaces glide over each other, e.g. acromo-clavicular joint.

Ball and socket joints — flexion, extension, abduction, adduction, rotation, circumduction, e.g. shoulder, hip.

Pivot joints — rotation round one axis only, e.g. atlas and axis.

Condyloid and saddle joint — movement round two axes allowing circumduction. e.g. wrist joint.

h Skeletal (or striped or striated or voluntary)

Smooth (or plain or visceral or involuntary)

Cardiac

i Irritability — ability to respond to a stimulus

Conductivity — convey an impulse

Extensibility — be stretched

Elasticity — resume original length

Contractility — shorten, thicken.

j **Movement** including breathing, mastication, facial expression, some sphincter control.

Maintenance of posture

Heat production Involuntary shivering.

Protection Prolonged tension in muscles 'warns' the patient that something is wrong — can be a diagnostic aid.

k Skeletal muscle is attached to the skeleton either directly or indirectly. The **origin** of the muscle is usually at the more fixed point and the **insertion** at the more mobile part.

Skeletal muscles, with the exception of the sphincter muscles, are attached to these origins and insertions by **white fibrous tissue** which may be rounded when it is called a **tendon** or may be a flattened sheet when it is called an **aponeurosis.**

l Each skeletal **muscle fibre** is supplied by a corresponding **nerve fibre** (which is a branch of the axon of a nerve cell which is situated in the anterior horn of the spinal cord) which ends as a flattened expansion. The muscle fibre has a corresponding structure known as a **motor end plate.** The small gap between the end of the motor nerve and the motor end plate of the muscle is called the **neuromuscular junction.**

m As the nerve impulse passes to the neuromuscular junction acetylcholine is released which 'bridges the gap', stimulates electrical changes in the end plate, thus causing contraction of the muscle fibre. **Acetylcholine** is destroyed by **cholinesterase,** an enzyme found in the muscle at the end plates.

n Muscle tone is a state of continuous partial contraction maintained by groups of muscle cells contracting in relays. Thus, even when muscle appears to be at rest, it is always partially contracted and therefore ready for immediate action. It is the degree and distribution of this tone that determines body posture.

o A cross-section of the spinal cord shows a central H-shaped grey area which consists of nerve cells. The white area around the H consists of nerve fibres. The H-shaped grey matter is described as having two anterior horns and two posterior horns. The cells of origin of the motor nerves are found in the anterior horns, each anterior horn cell gives rise to a single axon which leaves via the anterior nerve root.

p Every anterior horn cell innervates many muscle fibres. Each anterior horn cell gives rise to a single axon. When the axon reaches the muscle, it branches and supplies a group of voluntary muscle fibres. Thus, the anterior horn cell, the axon and its branches and all the muscle fibres supplied by the same anterior horn cell are collectively termed a **motor unit.**

q When a muscle shortens and produces movement but the tension remains the same, the contraction is termed **isotonic.** When the tension of the muscle increases but the length of the muscle remains the same the contraction is termed **isometric.**

r The sensory cortex is the area of the cerebrum which lies behind the central sulcus (fissure of Rolando). Sensory impulses from one side of the body are received and interpreted in the sensory cortex in the opposite hemisphere.

s An afferent or sensory nerve has its cell of origin in the spinal ganglia which lie outside the spinal cord in the posterior nerve root. These sensory nerves have receptors in the skin and deeper structures from where they convey information into the spinal cord via the posterior nerve roots. (From here the impulse is transmitted via sensory pathways to the sensory cortex of the brain.)

t A reflex action is an automatic motor response to a sensory stimulus that occurs without conscious initiation. The individual usually becomes aware of the reflex activity after it has occurred because the impulses eventually reaching the sensory cortex are interpreted as sensation. Reflex actions are usually protective in function.

2

a Loss of muscular power due to interference with the nervous system, the muscle loses its ability to contract.

b The upper motor neurone refers to the neurone that constitutes the descending motor pathway from the cerebral cortex to the motor nuclei of the brainstem or the anterior horn of the spinal cord. A lesion at this level leads to spasticity of the muscles and reduced motor power.

c The lower motor neurone refers to the neurone that commences at the anterior horn cell in the spinal cord, or the motor cranial nerve nucleus in the brainstem and the axons. A lesion at this level leads to flaccidity, paralysis and atrophy of the muscle.

d A psychomotor defect in which there is an inability to use an object properly in spite of knowing its name and being able to describe its function, a loss of power to carry out regulated movements.

e Refers to the mechanism which gives us our sense of position and movement and by which we are able to adjust our muscular movements to a great degree of accuracy and to maintain our equilibrium. This is brought about by sensory nerve impulses from receptors called proprioceptors — these include muscle spindles, tendon and organs, joint receptors and vestibular receptors.

f Placing the limbs in the most favourable position, usually the most natural position of slight flexion.

g Weakness of the dorsiflexors of the foot and toes which causes an inability to raise the front part of the foot from the ground or in which, when the condition is severe, the foot hangs limp. It can follow damage to the anterior tibial nerve and may also be a complication of bedrest if preventative measures are not taken.

h Refers to exercises which the patient is able to carry out himself.

i Refers to exercises in which the patient does not play an active part, e.g. the limbs may be put through a full range of movement by the physiotherapist or nurse.

j Osteoporosis means increased porousness of the bone and softening due to lack of calcium salts. Can be due to the ageing process but is also a complication of prolonged periods of immobilisation in bed.

k Wasting or shrinkage in the size of the muscle. It can be caused by diminished function through long periods of immobilisation, by joint disorders, circulatory disturbance, continuous pressure and lower motor neurone disease. It results in a reduction of muscle power.

l The formation of a blood clot in the deep veins (usually of the leg). It is associated with congestive heart failure, immobilisation, varicose veins and appears to be a complication of advanced malignant disease. Venous thrombosis tends to complicate surgery.

m Dystrophy means defective or faulty nutrition and refers to changes in the muscles occurring independently of the nervous system. There may be atrophic or hypertrophic changes associated with loss of power.

n An abnormal sensation such as burning, itching, prickling, numbness.

3
a	xi or xiii	**f**	iv	**k**	xiv
b	vi	**g**	viii	**l**	i or ii
c	vii	**h**	xii	**m**	iii
d	vi or viii	**i**	x	**n**	i or ii
e	ix	**j**	v		

13 ADVICE FOR EXAMINATION PREPARATION

Start your preparation well in advance of the examination. Make a realistic plan of action that you will be able to achieve.

1 Decide how many hours each day you can set aside for study/revision. 2 hours daily × 5 = 10 hours weekly.
2 Make a timetable and slot in all the subjects to be studied. The length of time you allocate depends on the level of difficulty.
3 Study in the same place each day. Sit at a desk or table and have the materials you need at hand i.e. paper, pencils, crayons, text books, lecture notes and a rubber. Write in pencil so that mistakes or unwanted notes can be erased (paper is expensive).
4 You must work at concentrating on your task, don't allow yourself to think of anything else so that you waste time.
5 If you are tired or upset, relax before attempting to settle.
6 Work at each of the goals you have set yourself as widely as you can.
7 Reward yourself when a goal is achieved so that you associate pleasure with studying.
8 Success is not a matter of luck but of good planning and self-discipline.
9 Learning is an active process so:
  a Study using a logical appraoch. Sequence the material and go from easy to more difficult concepts.
  b Don't try to learn chunks of material, skim the passage and try to understand. Underline key words or sentences. Use a dictionary.
  c Overlearn material and consciously recall and reinforce your memory. Commit your thoughts to paper.
  d Use mnemonics as a memory aid.
  e Ask yourself questions, apply the material, compare with management of actual patients you have nursed. Have discussions with friends/tutors.
  f Ask your tutors for help if you do not understand the relevance of a topic.
  g Learn to draw and label line drawings correctly.
  h Test yourself using past examination questions.
  i Get your relations or friends to ask you questions.
10 Cultivate a fast reading style. Use several textbooks with your notes. Make your own notes when you have analysed the meaning of a passage. Begin to read with a question in mind and ask yourself

questions when you have read a paragraph/chapter. Read quickly then re-read.

11 What you want to achieve is efficiency of study with economy of effort.

Examination technique

1 Listen to the Invigilator's instructions and follow them carefully. Have your number card signed and available for inspection. Be prepared with pens, pencils, a rubber and ruler.

2 Read the instructions on the front cover of the book and comply with them i.e. start a question on a fresh page, number your questions carefully, write legibly. Note how many questions are to be attempted, how much time is allowed etc.

3 Objective type questions test a wide area of knowledge, recognition and recall in a short time. Consider the questions carefully, and choose what you believe to be the correct answer from the distractors, do not just guess.

4 Essay questions test:
   a Knowledge
   b Comprehension
   c Application
   d Communication
   e Synthesis.

5 Read all the questions carefully on both sides of the paper, identify all parts of the question and answer either/or type.
   a Don't be concerned that others have started to write.
   b Select the questions you feel most able to answer.
   c Tick your selection in order of sequence.
   d Analyse the setting of the question. Is the scene in hospital or the community? What is the importance of age, sex, marital/social status, environment, psychological well-being, needs of the patient in the examiner's mind. Underline these points and develop them.
   e Note the essential points that have to be made in your answer in the margin of the paper.
   f Pay attention to the weighting of each part of the question, these should help you plan the time to be spent on each part.
   g Ten minutes spent in planning is the most effective way of using the examination time.
   h When you start to write:
      i Answer the parts in order of a, b, c, d.
      ii Write legibly, be logical (first things first).
      iii Concentrate on the main parts, don't waffle and repeat yourself.

    iv   If a diagram is asked for, make a clear line drawing and label it clearly.

    v   Leave time at the end for reading your answers.

Remember that a good essay has an introduction, a development and a conclusion, and should be clear and concise.

NOTES

NOTES

NOTES

Exams?

Nurses don't have much time to study and revise. Which is why the study you can do has to count – has to be the *right* kind of study.

Celtic Revision Aids can help. With the new Celtic Revision Aids **Nursing Revision Notes** series, you can make the best of your training, by organising your study and revision properly, learning the *right* facts and the *right* way to apply them on the ward, and the *right* exam technique. The **Nursing Revision Notes** series is the *right* range for you, because the books are designed as a series of single subject practical nursing modules for use all the way through your course *and* in the vital revision period before your exams.

The **Nursing Revision Notes** series covers the most up-to-date syllabus requirements and will build rapidly into a complete set of titles for every subject you'll have to study during your nursing training.

Every title in the **Nursing Revision Notes** series is written by qualified and practising Nursing Tutors and Examiners — so you know that you're in the *right* hands!

Get it right!

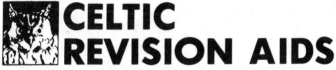

Principles of Nursing   £1.95
This title takes the learner through, in detail, the nurse's responsibilities from the time of the patient's admission until discharge. The emphasis is on nursing care: nursing observations, the nurse's role in investigations, and ideas on how the nurse can help the patient overcome the various problems of hospitalization. Each chapter is finished by practice examination questions. The final chapter contains advice on examination preparation.

General Medical Nursing   £1.95
The introductory chapter defines the general principles of nursing care which apply for the nursing of all patients being treated for common medical conditions. Successive chapters deal with specific diseases and explain the disease process, the management of the disease, and the specific nursing care. At the end of each chapter are examination style questions, to test the learner's understanding of the material. The final chapter contains advice on examination preparation.

Surgical Nursing   £1.95
This book begins by defining the general principles of nursing care which apply in pre- and post- operative stages. The following chapters deal with different parts of the anatomy, explaining symptoms, investigations, surgery, and treatment that the patient with common problems needing surgical intervention will experience. Again, the emphasis is on nursing care in the surgical situation and, again, each chapter ends with a section of practice examination questions for nurse learners to test their understanding of the chapter. The final chapter contains advice on examination preparation.

Other books to be published in this series over the next two years are: *Paediatric Nursing; Ear, Nose and Throat Nursing; Ophthalmic Nursing; Orthopaedic Nursing; Obstetric and Gynaecological Nursing; Psychiatric Nursing; Geriatric and Psychogeriatric Nursing.*